Tackling health inequalities since the Acheson Inquiry

Mark Exworthy, Marian Stuart, David Blane and Michael Marmot

The POLICY PRESS

499000979

First published in Great Britain in March 2003 by

The Policy Press
Fourth Floor, Beacon House
Queen's Road
Bristol BS8 1QU
UK

Tel no +44 (0)117 331 4054
Fax no +44 (0)117 331 4093
E-mail tpp-info@bristol.ac.uk
www.policypress.org.uk

© University College London 2003

Published for the Joseph Rowntree Foundation by The Policy Press

ISBN 1 86134 504 6

Mark Exworthy was formerly Senior Research Fellow at the International Centre for Health and Society, Department of Epidemiology and Public Health, University College London, **Marian Stuart** is an independent consultant, **David Blane** is Reader in the Department of Primary Care and Population Health Sciences, Imperial College London and **Michael Marmot** is Director of the International Centre for Health and Society, Department of Epidemiology and Public Health, University College London.

The **Joseph Rowntree Foundation** has supported this project as part of its programme of research and innovative development projects, which it hopes will be of value to policy makers, practitioners and service users. The facts presented and views expressed in this report are, however, those of the authors and not necessarily those of the Foundation.

The statements and opinions contained within this publication are solely those of the authors and contributors and not of The University of Bristol or The Policy Press. The University of Bristol and The Policy Press disclaim responsibility for any injury to persons or property resulting from any material published in this publication.

The Policy Press works to counter discrimination on grounds of gender, race, disability, age and sexuality.

Cover design by Qube Design Associates, Bristol
Photograph on front cover kindly supplied by www.third-avenue.co.uk
Printed in Great Britain by Hobbs the Printers Ltd, Southampton

Contents

Acknowledgements

This project was funded by the Joseph Rowntree Foundation. We are grateful for their support and especially the assistance and advice of Pat Kneen.

The project was supported by an Advisory Group, the members of which provided most helpful, constructive comments. The members of this Group are listed in Appendix A. Civil servants from many departments contributed their time and ideas to the work of this project; their advice was particularly constructive.

Foreword

When in May 1997 I was invited by Tessa Jowell, then Secretary of State for Health, "to review and summarise inequalities in health in England and to identify priority areas for policies to reduce them", I had good reason to be sceptical whether anything would come of it. While the work would obviously require an extended effort on my part, I knew from my personal experience of Whitehall, that Ministerial enthusiasms may be evanescent, and often evaporate in the next shuffle. Even worse, as had happened to my distinguished predecessor Sir Douglas Patrick, a report commissioned by one government may be ignored or even suppressed by its successor.

But, as things turned out, an apparently inconsequential breach of protocol on Tessa's part was to dispel my concerns. Having recruited me to chair the Inquiry, Tessa briefed the press having forgotten to inform the Prime Minister first. What words passed between them I do not know, but the outcome was most advantageous. On 11 June 1997, in an arranged Parliamentary Question put to Tony Blair, the matter was rectified, and our Report was provided with unassailable support for at least as long as the government was in power:

> ... it is for this reason that the Secretary of State for Health has asked Sir Donald Acheson to conduct a further review of inequalities in health. Those inequalities do matter and there is no doubt that the published statistics show a link between income inequality and poor health.

The Independent Inquiry held its first meeting in September 1997 and its report was published almost exactly a year later. Our approach was based on a socioeconomic explanation of health inequalities. This tracks the roots of ill-health

widely to such determinants as income, education and employment, as well as to the material environment and lifestyle. Such a model of course carries the implication that remedial action must be a responsibility of the whole government and is by no means exclusively a matter for the Department of Health, let alone the National Health Service.

That this point is now fully understood and accepted became clear last year when, as part of the current 'cross-cutting spending review' chaired by HM Treasury, a gathering of officials from all government departments met together in Whitehall to consider their policies under the title 'Tackling health inequalities'.

Nevertheless, in the midst of those well-directed political aspirations, social science has a further crucial contribution to make, if these aspirations are to be realised. Hence the timely value of this report. As Mark Exworthy correctly points out, in the Independent Inquiry Report, having set out our view of the *ends*, in the shape of three priority areas and 74 recommendations, we gave little or no guidance about the *means* by which these ends would be achieved. This report fills that gap. It contains a wealth of practical suggestions about developments in processes and systems, which are essential if the reduction of inequalities is to become a reality. It provides a toolbox that must be given a permanent place in the mechanics of bureaucracy if the obstinate trend seen throughout the last century is to be reversed.

Donald Acheson

List of useful acronyms

ACRA	Advisory Committee on Resource Allocation
CAP	Common Agricultural Policy
CASE	Centre for Analysis of Social Exclusion
CHD	coronary heart disease
CSR	Comprehensive Spending Review
DA(SER)	Domestic Affairs Sub-Committee on Social Exclusion and Regeneration (the Secretary of State for Work and Pensions, and the Chief Secretary to the Treasury are members of the Committee)
DCMS	Department for Culture, Media and Sport
DEFRA	Department for Environment, Food and Rural Affairs (formerly part of the DETR and MAFF)
DETR	Department of the Environment, Transport and the Regions
DfEE	Department for Education and Employment
DfES	Department for Education and Skills
DfT	Department for Transport
DoH	Department of Health
DPH	Directors of Public Health
DSS	Department of Social Security
DTI	Department of Trade and Industry
DTLR	Department for Transport, Local Government and the Regions
DWP	Department for Work and Pensions (formerly the DfEE and DSS)
ESRC	Economic and Social Research Council
EU	European Union
EYDCP	Early Years Development and Childcare Plan
HA	health authority
HAZ	Health Action Zone
HDA	Health Development Agency
HImP	Health Improvement Programme
HLC	healthy living centre
HMT	Her Majesty's Treasury

ICC	Integrated Child Credit
ICT	information and communication technologies
IFS	Institute for Fiscal Studies
IMR	infant mortality rate
JRF	Joseph Rowntree Foundation
LA	local authority
LEA	local education authority
LSP	local strategic partnership
MAFF	Ministry of Agriculture, Fisheries and Food
MRC	Medical Research Council
NAO	National Audit Office
NHS	National Health Service
NICE	National Institute for Clinical Excellence
NMW	national minimum wage
NRU	Neighbourhood Renewal Unit
NSF	National Service Framework
ODPM	Office of the Deputy Prime Minister
OECD	Organisation for Economic Co-operation and Development
ONS	Office for National Statistics
PAT	Policy Action Team (within the Cabinet Office)
PCT	primary care trust
PIU	Performance and Innovation Unit (part of the SEU)
PSA	public service agreement
SAFF	service and financial framework
SDA	service delivery agreement
SEU	Social Exclusion Unit
STAG	School Travel Advisory Group
StHA	Strategic Health Authority
UCL	University College London
WFTC	Working Families' Tax Credit (from April 2003 the WFTC will become the WTC)
WTC	Working Tax Credit
YOT	youth offending team

Introduction

Aims

This report reviews the progress made by the government, its agencies and others to implement the recommendations of the Independent Inquiry into Inequalities in Health. The report also examines the ways in which the UK government has sought to formulate and implement policies to tackle health inequalities. More broadly, themes and issues that are emerging from policy implementation are also considered.

The Labour government and the Inquiry marked three significant changes in national policy towards health inequalities in the UK. First, commissioned soon after the general election in May 1997, the Inquiry signalled that health inequalities were recognised as a legitimate 'problem' by government. This marked a change from previous administrations. However, while much is known about the causes and manifestations of health inequalities (Graham, 2000) and the wider determinants of health (Marmot and Wilkinson, 1999), relatively little is known about how policies can tackle them. Second, the Inquiry formed part of a wider approach to tackling inequality and social exclusion across government (Powell, 1999). Third, the Inquiry denoted the Labour government's approach of 'what counts is what works' and thereby indicated a new relationship between research and policy (Davies et al, 2000).

Methodology

Commissioned in July 1997 and published in November 1998, the Inquiry occurred during the first 18 months of the first term of the Labour government. This research project began in February 2001, shortly before the June 2001 general election that returned the Labour government for a second term. The research identified policy developments up to and including *Tackling health inequalities: A summary of the 2002 Cross-cutting Review*, published in November 2002 (see HM Treasury/DoH, 2002). The project therefore captured policy developments relating to the Inquiry and to health inequalities about 2½-4 years after the publication of the Inquiry. The research was also contemporaneous with ongoing policy developments.

The research was divided into two phases. The first phase (April-September 2001) 'mapped' policy action by each of the Inquiry's 74 recommendations. An initial search of policy documents identified a broad association between recommendation and policies. Individuals from departments were then invited to clarify or add to this mapping exercise. Responses were integrated. The second phase (October 2001-May 2002) involved case studies of contrasting areas of policy making relevant to health inequalities. Case studies thus enabled a closer inspection of policies relevant to health inequalities while providing a spectrum across different policy sectors. They represented key aspects of current policies to tackle health inequalities that might reveal broader themes for ongoing and future policy development. The case studies (tax and benefit reform, performance management, and transport) explored the nature of the problem, policy developments and evidence of progress thus far. Issues such as joined-up government, the application of a social gradient in policy making, the monitoring of policy, and policy approaches across the life span, were examined. Data included official documents, informal interviews with 32 civil servants, and commentaries and evaluations.

Policy research such as this is liable to becoming quickly out of date as new policies and programmes are developed. While the study has been careful to avoid this through close collaboration with government departments, the 'perishable' nature of this evidence underlines the need for wider perspectives and interpretation (see Chapter 6). This approach aids a more analytical view and considers broad themes running through various policies.

The research was conducted in the International Centre for Health and Society in the Department of Epidemiology and Public Health at University College London (UCL). Sir Donald Acheson held the chairmanship of the International Centre at the time of the Independent Inquiry. Management of the Inquiry was shared by the Secretariat (comprising three people) and the Scientific Advisory Group (comprising five people, and of whom only Professor Sir Michael Marmot was based at UCL). Bias was minimised as the researcher (Exworthy) and the policy advisor (Stuart) had been recruited from outside UCL and were not involved in the Inquiry's deliberations. The research was supported by an Advisory Group, which met five times (see Appendix A).

Independent Inquiry into Inequalities in Health

The Inquiry was commissioned in July 1997 with the following terms of reference:

1. To moderate a Department of Health review of the latest available information on inequalities in health, using data from the Office for National Statistics, the Department of Health and elsewhere. The data review would summarise the evidence of inequalities in health and expectation of life in England and identify trends.
2. In the light of that evidence, to conduct – within the broad framework of the Government's overall financial strategy – an independent review to identify priority areas for future policy

development, which scientific and expert evidence indicates are likely to offer opportunities for Government to develop beneficial, cost-effective and affordable interventions to reduce health inequalities.
3. The review will report to the Secretary of State for Health. The report will be published and its conclusion, based on evidence, will contribute to the development of a new strategy for health. (Acheson, 1998, p iv)

Drawing on 'input papers' on 17 areas (including policy sectors, social groups and disease categories) and published evidence, the Inquiry team (see Appendix B) concluded that the "weight of scientific evidence supports a socio-economic explanation of health inequalities" (p xi). Overall, there were 39 main recommendations (see Appendix C) but most had subsidiary recommendations (which totalled 74). Three recommendations were highlighted in the report's synopsis as being "crucial":

1. all policies likely to have an impact on health should be evaluated in terms of their impact on health inequalities;
2. a high priority should be given to the health of families with children;
3. further steps should be taken to reduce income inequalities and improve the living standards of poor households (p xi).

The government "welcomed" the report and indicated that it was already implementing many of the recommended policies (DoH, 1998a). A few months later, an 'action report' on tackling health inequalities was published at the same time as the public health White Paper, *Saving lives: Our healthier nation* (DoH, 1999a), which drew heavily on the Inquiry's report.

Many academics and practitioners supported the Inquiry's report, but five critiques can be identified:

* no priorities among the recommendations;
* no mechanisms or processes to expedite the recommendations;
* evidence did not always match the recommendations;

- recommendations ranged from the general to the specific; and
- economic evidence and perspectives were lacking (Exworthy, 2002).

Outline of this report

This report is divided into three main sections. Chapter 2 describes the policy context with emphasis on the content and chronology of current policies. Chapters 3, 4 and 5 present the three case studies, focusing on policy developments in contrasting sectors. Chapters 6 and 7 discuss the emergent themes from the empirical evidence, consider interpretations of progress and offer recommendations for future policy making.

2

Policy context, content and chronology

This chapter examines the context, the chronology and content of specific policies related to health inequalities.

Policy context and evolution

In dealing with health inequalities, the inimical political climate since the 'Black Report' (Black, 1980) effectively stifled national initiatives (Berridge and Blume, 2002). Nonetheless, many local agencies had pursued their own strategies. This context began to shift during the mid-1990s with the introduction of the term of 'health variations'; in 1994, the Department of Health (DoH) established a committee to explore 'social variations in health'. The terminology was significant – 'variations' did not carry the same meaning as 'inequalities' but the term was a tacit recognition that they posed a policy problem.

The election of the Labour government in May 1997 provided a major transition in policy, as health inequalities became a formal component of the government's programme and health inequalities were an explicit part of the agenda of central government. The term 'inequalities' was back in favour. Table 2.1 illustrates the policy programme from 1997.

However, the incoming government accepted the spending plans of the previous government for the first three years, thereby limiting the (fiscal) scope of initiatives. Policy was still dominated by the wider structures and processes of government and socioeconomic forces.

Key policy developments

Defining those policies that are related to efforts to tackle health inequalities can be problematic. Hence, the key developments, summarised below, are inevitably selective.

The Green Paper *Our healthier nation* (DoH, 1998b) was a follow-up to the first strategy for health (*Health of the nation*; DoH, 1992). Its aim was to improve the health of the population as a whole and to improve the health of the worst off in society. The strategy included a 'contract for health' between government, public agencies and the public in order to meet their responsibilities for health. Four targets were proposed, covering heart disease and stroke, accidents, cancer and mental health.

The White Paper *Saving lives: Our healthier nation* (DoH, 1999a) was the first major health strategy published after the Acheson Report. It drew on the Acheson Report by emphasising the need to reduce health inequalities. It also confirmed the health targets originally proposed in the Green Paper but did not set health inequality targets, leaving these to local discretion (the Scottish White Paper [Scottish Office, 1999] placed a greater emphasis on targets).

An *Action report* on reducing health inequalities (DoH, 1999b) was published at the same time as the White Paper. It accepted the findings of the Acheson Report and referred to policies for a fairer society, building healthy communities, education, employment, housing, transport, crime and healthcare. It also reported on the appointment of a Public Health Minister, Public Health White Paper, Smoking White Paper, the Independent Inquiry and a refocusing of healthcare provision.

Table 2.1: Selected policy 'events' applicable to tackling health inequalities in the UK

1980	*Inequalities in health* report (Black Report) published
1985	*Targets for health for all* published (by WHO)
1995	*Variations in health: What can the Department of Health and NHS do?* published
1995	*Review of the research on the effectiveness of health service interventions to reduce variations in health* published (Centre for Reviews and Dissemination, York).
May 1997	Labour government elected
	Tessa Jowell appointed as Minister of Public Health
July 1997	Independent Inquiry into Inequalities in Health commissioned
December 1997	*The new NHS: Modern, dependable* published
February 1998	*Our healthier nation: A contract for health* Green Paper (Cmd 3852) published
November 1998	Independent Inquiry into Inequalities in Health (Acheson Report) published
April 1999	*New NHS* arrangements come into force
	Primary Care Groups established
June 1999	Health Act passed
July 1999	*Saving lives: Our healthier nation* White Paper (Cmd 4386) published
	Local targets for reducing health inequalities
	Reducing health inequalities: An action report published
September 1999	First National Service Framework (mental health) published
	Opportunity for all – Tackling poverty and social exclusion published with the aim to eradicate child poverty in 20 years
October 1999	Yvette Cooper appointed as Parliamentary Under Secretary for Public Health; Ministerial responsibilities include health inequalities
November 1999	Sure Start programme begins
January 2000	*Wiring it up* report published (Cabinet Office)
July 2000	*The NHS Plan* published
	National health inequalities targets to be introduced
	Public service agreements (*2000 Spending Review*) published (HM Treasury)
Autumn 2000	Inequalities and public health taskforce established
January 2001	*A new commitment to neighbourhood renewal: National strategy action plan* published (SEU)
February 2001	National health inequalities targets announced
March 2001	Health Select Committee inquiry into public health published
June 2001	General election; Labour returned for second term
	A cross-cutting review on health inequalities announced as part of the *2002 Spending Review*
July 2001	*Shifting the balance of power: Securing delivery* – giving PCTs new powers; creating Strategic Health Authorities; and reducing the DoH's direct management role
	Government's response to the Health Select Committee report on public health (Cm 5242) published
August 2001	DoH *From vision to reality* document published
	DoH *Tackling health inequalities: Consultation on a plan for delivery* starts
Nov 2001	DoH *Tackling health inequalities: Consultation of a plan for delivery* ends
	Wanless (interim) Report (*Securing our future health*) published
March 2002	*Tackling health inequalities: Update* published
April 2002	Wanless (final) Report (*Securing our future health*) published
June 2002	Hazel Blears appointed as Minister for Public Health (replacing Yvette Cooper)
	DoH *Consultation on a plan for delivery* published
July 2002	*2002 Spending Review: New public spending plans 2003-2006* published (HM Treasury)
October 2002	*Health and neighbourhood renewal: Guidance from the Department of Health and the Neighbourhood Renewal Unit* published
November 2002	*Tackling health inequalities: A summary of the 2002 Cross-cutting Review* published (HM Treasury/DoH)

Note: For a similar chronology of Labour's welfare reform, see Powell, 1999, pp 40-1.

The NHS Plan (DoH, 2000) focused largely on healthcare, but Chapter 13 ('Improving health and reducing inequalities') summarised government actions for health inequalities:

* setting a national health inequalities target;
* reducing inequalities in access to NHS services;
* children: ensuring a healthy start in life;
* reducing smoking;
* improving diet and nutrition;
* tackling drugs and alcohol-related crime; and
* new partnerships to tackle inequality. (pp 106-11)

The national targets for health inequalities (which were prefigured in *The NHS Plan*) were announced in February 2001, focusing on infant mortality and life expectancy.

Starting with children under one year, by 2010, to reduce by at least 10% the gap in mortality between manual groups and the population as a whole.

Starting with health authorities, by 2010, to reduce by at least 10% the gap between the fifth of areas with the lowest life expectancy at birth and the population as a whole. (p iii)

The infant mortality rate for England and Wales fell to 5.6 deaths per 1,000 live births in 2000 (from 5.8 in 1999); however, the gap between manual social groups and the general population widened by 0.5% between 1997-99 and 1998-2000 (DoH, 2002a). Life expectancy for women in England was 80.2 years and 75.4 years for men in 1998-2000. The difference in life expectancy between the lowest fifth of areas and the national average has not changed in recent years, but the gap between the 'best' and 'worst' areas grew to 6.6. years for women and 7.7 years for men (DoH, 2002a).

From vision to reality (DoH, 2001a) summarised the initiatives that the government had introduced or were planning to implement. It outlined the public health policies, many of which had previously been highlighted by *The NHS Plan* and which were being overseen by the Inequalities and Public Health Taskforce (p 2). The report addressed:

* action against the big killers (cancer, coronary heart disease and mental health);
* joining forces to make things happen...; and
* strengthening the evidence base.

In August 2001, the DoH published *Tackling health inequalities: Consultation on a plan for delivery* (2001b), which invited views on the national targets for health inequalities. The document summarised six priorities (pregnancy and childhood, children and young people, primary care, tackling coronary heart disease [CHD] and cancer, aiding deprived communities, tackling wider determinants). The results of the consultation were published in June 2002 (DoH, 2002b), reporting that consultation responses called for national action in terms of:

* more robust mechanisms for funding allocation across the public sector;
* a shift from short-term project funding to mainstream budgets; and
* better systems for bidding against remaining initiatives. (p 22)

Further suggestions were made in relation to training, joint appointments, "better integrated planning systems, consistent performance management across sectors, and targets between national, regional and local government" (p 24). Following the consultation results and the Comprehensive Spending Review (HM Treasury, 2002), a delivery plan was published in autumn 2002. The plan was intended to be "evidence-based ..., set out a cross-government strategy for health inequalities ... and ensure[d] that local delivery systems are not over-burdened" (p 27).

In June 2001, the second round of cross-cutting reviews included health inequalities. The review comprised two elements: developing an evidence base and forming a strategy for delivery. In the *2002 Spending Review* (HM Treasury, 2002) a two-page summary of the cross-cutting review drew on the Independent Inquiry and the Wanless Report (Wanless, 2002). It also highlighted the range of current strategies and identified the "need for long-term government-wide strategy to ensure that health inequalities objectives are reflected in departments' mainstream programmes" (HM Treasury, 2002, p 157). Recommendations included:

- stronger focus on deprived areas in the allocation of resources for the NHS and schools;
- better preventative health care services for disadvantaged communities [including an expansion of smoking cessation services];
- targeted services for disadvantaged communities [including a focus on children's nutrition];
- expansion of initiatives to raise levels of physical activity in disadvantaged communities; and
- improved housing conditions for families with young children and for elderly people. (p 158)

The review also focused on "improving the coordination and targeting of mainstream public services". The implementation of the review's long-term strategy will be overseen by a Ministerial committee.

Tackling health inequalities: A summary of the 2002 Cross-cutting Review was published in November 2002 (HM Treasury/DoH, 2002). This covered:

- a long-term strategy for tackling health inequalities;
- the top priorities for meeting national health inequality targets;
- key themes of the review;
- delivering the health inequalities strategy; and
- a supporting analysis of the problem, causes and risk factors.

It included a comprehensive analysis of the problem, which endorsed the findings of the Inquiry's Report, and a clear commitment to pursue a long-term strategy to tackle health inequalities and the wider determinants of health. In the introduction to the document Hazel Blears affirmed that "Tackling health inequalities is a top priority for this Government" (p v).

The document provided welcome recognition that health inequalities follow a social gradient and that interventions need to reach more than the most deprived areas and the most disadvantaged in order to make progress. It set out a strategy for health inequalities that includes:

- the context of government action (the child poverty strategy, the Local Government White Paper, *Strong local leadership* (DTLR, 2001a) and so on);
- mainstreaming (in priority programmes for national and local government, in formulae for allocating resources and so on);
- breaking the cycle of health inequalities (reducing poverty, narrowing the gap in educational attainment and so on);
- tackling the major killers (through smoking cessation, diet, physical activity, reducing accidental injury, improved mental health and reduced work-related illness and injury);
- improving access to public services and facilities (improving access to primary care, levelling up access to preventive and treatment services, improving access to healthy and affordable food, improving public transport, making services more joined up);
- strengthening disadvantaged communities (neighbourhood renewal, tackling crime, improving housing and so on);
- supporting targeted interventions for specific groups (black and ethnic minorities, those with complex needs, older people, ending fuel poverty and so on);
- using information to support action (across a range of health dimensions, developing an evidence base and developing health inequalities impact assessment).

The report announced that a cross-government delivery plan to March 2006 is being developed, which will be taken forward by "proposed new Ministerial and official structures" (p 3). The DoH will be responsible for coordinating action to implement it; HM Treasury and the Prime Minister's Delivery Unit will monitor progress; and it will be overseen by the Cabinet's Domestic Affairs Sub-Committee on Social Exclusion and Regeneration (DA(SER)).

Structures and processes for tackling health inequalities

The Labour government has taken a more consultative approach to policy formulation, notably in the formation and use of taskforces. Barker et al (1999) identified the creation of 279 taskforces and 15 major inquiries in the first two years of the government – the Independent

Inquiry as one of the latter. Both taskforces and inquiries are marked by the inclusion of officials and external 'experts' or representatives into policy making. In addition, other, more standard structures and processes can also be identified (Table 2.2).

'Mainstreaming' policies to tackle health inequalities

Many policies relevant to tackling health inequalities have been new initiatives or projects limited to particular geographical areas and/or are time-limited. These can remain isolated from 'mainstream' planning processes and service delivery. Mainstream programmes will have to bear most responsibility for tackling health inequalities, as recognised by the *2002 Spending Review* (HM Treasury, 2002). Mainstreaming has been defined as:

> the application of learning and new behaviour into core activities of the organisation. (Maddock, 2000, p 1)

It also covers the achievement of core funding for pilots and projects. Three forms of mainstreaming have been identified (Stewart et al, 2002):

- *Projects:* Funding was secured to continue particular activities.
- *Good practice:* A (national or local) 'mainstream' agency "adapts and reproduces" examples of good practice from initiatives. Stewart and colleagues found little evidence of this form in area-based initiatives.
- *Policy:* Policy lessons from work and experience of initiatives have direct influence on the policy process.

A fourth form might involve the systems and processes to monitor and/or coordinate the development and outcomes of policies.

Mainstreaming will need to tackle the barriers identified in area-based initiatives such as Health Action Zones (HAZs) and Sure Start:

1. weak leadership is disconnected from internal culture issues;
2. initiatives remain detached from wider agendas;
3. attention is on 'early wins' and discrete output projects;
4. lack of organisational development and staff involvement champions;
5. lack of political steer;
6. implementation processes are "invisible" in plans or guidance;

Table 2.2: Examples of structures and processes relevant to tackling health inequalities

Inquiry/Royal Commission	Independent Inquiry into Inequalities in Health (Acheson Report)
Taskforce	Inequalities and Public Health Taskforce
	Children's Taskforce
	Policy Action Teams (SEU) (such as PAT 12: Young People and PAT 13: Improving shopping access)
Dedicated cross-departmental unit	Sure Start Unit
	Teenage Pregnancy Unit
	Children and Young People's Unit
	Neighbourhood Renewal Unit
	Social Exclusion Unit
Inter-departmental group (including steering or advisory groups)	Cross-Government Group on Public Health and Inequalities (DoH-led)
	2002 Cross-cutting Review on health inequalities (HM Treasury-led)
	Health Agenda Network (ODPM)
Resource allocation	Advisory Committee on Resource Allocation (DoH)
Performance management	National health inequalities targets
	National Framework for the Assessment of Performance
	Public services agreements and service delivery agreements
Consultation	DoH *Tackling health inequalities: Consultation on a plan for delivery*
	SEU reports (for example, on transport and social exclusion)
	Wanless Report

7. local stakeholders are "hesitant";
8. short-termism persists;
9. lack of organisational flexibility;
10. lack of innovation;
11. poor lesson learning (1-7: Maddock, 2000; 8-11: Stewart et al, 2002).

Ways to improve mainstreaming include:

1. more explicit evaluation to assess what works for the mainstream;
2. development of explicit continuity or forward (rather than exit) strategies;
3. more attention to and shared responsibility of exchange of experience between initiatives;
4. input from initiatives into mainstream planning processes and vice versa;
5. closer links at senior level between initiatives and mainstream policy or delivery agencies; and
6. linking initiatives directly into the achievement of mainstream targets (Stewart et al, 2002).

'National' mainstreaming of policies relevant to health inequalities is needed within the DoH and across government. Within the DoH, health inequalities could be seen as a discrete area of public health; key strategies (for example the NSF) must therefore take account of health inequalities and avoid them being overlooked in meeting other objectives such as waiting times. The dual approach of mainstreaming policies relevant to health inequalities and implementing key strategies needs to manage the tension between achieving reductions in mortality by the 'big killers' while skewing these targets to tackle health inequalities. If achieved, this approach could generate significant outcomes.

Beyond the DoH, policies related to health inequalities need to be funded on a long-term and secure basis, and their relevance given full recognition. The tensions between a department's core objectives and adjustments necessary to ensure inequalities are reduced (and not increased further) need to be recognised and addressed. Health inequalities may be seen as a 'health'/DoH issue, with little connection to other departmental strategies – where health inequalities have been addressed by other departments this has often permeated only a small way into mainstream planning processes.

The importance of mainstreaming was underlined by the report of the *2002 Cross-cutting Review* on health inequalities, which argued that:

- Tackling health inequalities should be mainstreamed within priority programmes and reflected within the formulation and implementation of the policies of national and local government "giving disproportionate benefit to those suffering material disadvantage or who have traditionally been poorly served".
- National health inequalities targets need to be embedded in and delivered through mainstream programmes across government.
- Formulae used by departments for allocating national resources should reflect the geographical distribution of need.
- Challenging floor targets should be set to 'level up' service quality and outcomes.
- Mechanisms should be developed to disseminate learning from successful local initiatives including Sure Start and Health Action Zones.
- Progress towards targets needs to be monitored and tracked using the cross-government basket of indicators and actively managed through performance assessment frameworks using local delivery targets and milestones.

Mapping current policies to tackle health inequalities

Current policies related to health inequalities were enumerated according to the Independent Inquiry's recommendations in a 'mapping exercise'. This was conducted in 2001 as the first phase of this project (see page 1) and monitoring has continued since. It found a significant amount of activity related to these policy objectives and most Inquiry recommendations, although some are certainly more developed than are others. Equally, there are additional policies that have been pursued but which were not recommended by the Independent Inquiry (such as health inequalities targets).

The mapping exercise identified the key departments currently most engaged in policies relevant to tackling health inequalities. These are the DoH, DfES, DWP, HM Treasury, DEFRA and the former DTLR (now the ODPM and DfT). The work of other departments (including the Home Office, DCMS and DTI) appears to be less closely targeted on or integrated with other strands of policy on health inequalities.

A selective description of the mapping exercise is presented under the headings used by the Acheson Report.

General: Recommendations 1 and 2

1. Health inequalities impact assessment
2. Priority to women of child-bearing age, expectant mothers and young children

The policy initiatives in this area have been patchy. Health inequalities impact assessment has not been widely adopted. Some departments (such as the former DTLR) established equality assessment procedures. Moreover, the data collection and monitoring processes surrounding health inequalities remain rather rudimentary (Recommendations 1.1, 1.2). However, the national health inequalities targets, the DoH consultation and the development of a 'basket' of indicators may ameliorate this. The 'gradient' of health inequalities, noted by the Health Select Committee's inquiry into public health, has only been partially incorporated, as 'social exclusion' has also been employed. The gradient assumes a relationship between lower incomes and poorer health across the entire population, while social exclusion denotes a binary division between 'excluded' and 'included' groups. Although much attention is focused on young children and women in pregnancy, there appears to be relatively little activity relating to women of childbearing age (Recommendation 2).

Poverty, income, tax and benefits: Recommendation 3

3. Income inequalities and living standards

The government set a target to 'eradicate' child poverty within a generation. To meet this target, it has introduced tax and benefit reforms, including benefit increases and tax credits, which are focused on low-income families with children. Tax credits underpin the government's approach, which involves linking welfare and employment strategies. A series of New Deals focus on specific population groups (such as

young people or disabled people) and seek to improve their (re-)entry into employment. Income-based minima have been introduced through the national minimum wage and the minimum income guarantee, yet these may be insufficient for a healthy living standard. Overall, these policies have been mildly redistributive across the social gradient but may be outweighed by rises in income inequalities.

Education: Recommendations 4-7

4. Additional resources for schools serving children from less well off groups
5. Pre-school education
6. Health promoting schools
7. Nutrition at school

Policies have focused on:

* educational attainment strategies;
* pre-school and nursery provision (such as provision of nursery school places for all three year olds from 2004);
* resource allocation formulae;
* health promoting schools (such as the National Healthy Schools Standard).

Probably the most significant policy initiative in this category is the Sure Start – a joint initiative between the DfES and DoH (Recommendation 4; see Chapter 4). Many Sure Start targets have an explicit health dimension, although health inequalities are largely implicit. Despite its recent expansion it does not cover all areas (focusing on areas of disadvantage) and will only cover a third of children in poverty (at its height).

Employment: Recommendations 8 and 9

8. Opportunities for work and ameliorating effects of unemployment
9. Quality of jobs and psychosocial work hazards

The government's priority has been to reduce unemployment and increase employment by increasing rates of employment (via various New Deal schemes and Action Teams for Jobs, for example; Recommendation 8) and by connecting welfare benefits much more closely to work incentives. These forms of work available should not exacerbate existing inequalities (in terms of, say, stress; Recommendation 9) and vulnerable groups should not be further disadvantaged in the process. Such initiatives have also been bolstered by attempts to raise living standards (through the national minimum wage; Recommendation 3). Furthermore, increases in Disability Living Allowance and Incapacity Benefit claims raise doubts about the overall effectiveness of employment initiatives.

Housing and environment: Recommendations 10-13

10. Availability of social housing
11. Housing provision and healthcare for homeless people
12. Quality of housing
13. Crime, violence and safe environments

Improvements to housing have fallen largely within the remit of the Neighbourhood Renewal Strategy (SEU, 2001) and the ODPM. Some specific initiatives fall within the remit of The Housing Corporation (Recommendation 10). The fuel poverty strategy (Recommendation 12.1) was published in November 2001 and involves an inter-Ministerial group, specific targets and financial support. Specifically, it involves winter fuel payments, a home energy efficiency scheme and decent homes standards for social housing (DWP, 2002a, p 121). Yet, the definition of vulnerable households will mean that there is a break-off point above which households do not benefit and hence is not specifically a 'gradient' approach. Finally, crime reduction is being tackled largely through 376 partnerships, mainly focused in areas of high deprivation (DWP, 2002a, p 121) (Recommendation 13).

Mobility, transport and pollution: Recommendations 14-18

14. Integration and affordability of public transport
15. Encouragement of walking and cycling, and separation of motor vehicles and others
16. Reduction in motor car usage
17. Reduction of traffic speed
18. Concessionary fares to older people and disadvantaged groups

Transport remains an area of policy initiatives that have yet to deliver fully (Recommendation 14; see Chapter 5). The 10-year plans are ambitious and will be affected by factors mainly

beyond the control of the government; their feasibility must therefore be questioned. For example, car usage has not fallen in recent years (Recommendation 16). However, strategies to meet the targets for reductions in traffic deaths and injuries (Recommendations 16 and 17), traffic-calming schemes, safety campaigns and school programmes have been introduced. Concessionary fares on public transport have been implemented in 94% of local authorities (DTLR, 2002) (Recommendation 18).

Nutrition and the Common Agricultural Policy: Recommendations 19 and 20

19. Review of the Common Agricultural Policy
20. Availability and affordability of food for a healthy diet

Previous government initiatives have stumbled over reform of the Common Agricultural Policy (Recommendation 19). However, current initiatives have been closely linked to 'healthy schools' programmes and some work has begun with the food industry on diet (Recommendation 20.2). The five-a-day programme comprises several aspects that encourage consumption of fruit and vegetables as part of a healthy diet. The National School Fruit Scheme (providing fruit to each child each school day) links health, education and nutrition strategies (Recommendation 7) and, following pilot schemes, it is being implemented gradually and will be rolled out nationally by 2004.

Mothers, children and families: Recommendations 21-23

21. Poverty in families with children
22. Health and nutrition of women of childbearing age
23. Social and emotional support for parents and children

The focus on children is emphasised in the Inquiry and this has been noted by government policy. The recommendations draw on areas such as Sure Start, education and diet. Reducing child poverty lies at the centre of current government policy (Recommendation 21), to be achieved through, for example, New Deals, tax credits and up-rating other benefits. Evidence shows that some progress is being made. However, those children being lifted out of poverty are living in households closest to the 'poverty line'; policy may find it difficult to affect those remaining in poverty. Households unaffected by welfare-to-work incentives will be most poorly affected. Moreover, child poverty reductions are complicated by rising income inequalities and the changing distribution of incomes. Connecting education and work, the childcare initiatives seek to reduce the gap between Sure Start areas and the rest of the country (Recommendation 21.1). This is one of the few examples to explicitly mention the gap or inequality. Fluoridation of water (Recommendation 22.2) has not been implemented. As the Health Select Committee noted, over half of health authorities have asked water companies to do so; none has complied. Health visiting services are being redeveloped (Recommendation 23.1) but it is unclear whether such professional development will necessarily involve a greater number of home visits.

Young people and adults of working age: Recommendations 24-26

24. Suicide among young people
25. Sexual health among young people and teenage pregnancy
26. Healthier lifestyles

Sexual health strategies are evident in the national strategy for sexual health and HIV (2001), the teenage conception rate target (see Chapter 4), local teenage pregnancy strategies and in the appointment of local teenage pregnancy coordinators (Recommendation 25). Healthier lifestyles (Recommendation 26) have traditionally been easier to adopt in more affluent groups, thereby widening health inequalities. It is not yet evident whether government efforts to tackle the 'major killers' (such as CHD) can or will address the social gradient with sufficient vigour. Evidence of smoking (especially among women) shows how some earlier policies can have the effect of widening health inequalities. Efforts are now targeted on persistent smokers (Recommendation 26.2; also Recommendation 22.3). The recommendation for nicotine replacement therapy on prescription (Recommendation 26.4) has been adopted. However, initial monitoring reveals largely process indicators of smoking cessation; follow-up studies to test the impact on

health inequalities will be required to test the long-term impact of this policy approach.

Older people: Recommendations 27-30

27. Material well-being of older people
28. Quality of homes for older people
29. Maintenance of mobility, independence and social contacts
30. Accessibility and availability of health and social services

Action on tackling health inequalities among the older population has taken place across many areas but is relatively limited compared with other population groups. This may be because much attention has been focused on children and younger people. Many of these initiatives relate to standards of living (Recommendation 27) (benefit increase), such as the minimum income guarantee and above-inflation increases in the basic state pension (DWP, 2001, p 115). A campaign to encourage up-take in the minimum income guarantee has reduced the proportion of pensioners who live in a low-income household (from 27% in 1996/97 to 19% in 1999/2000, after housing costs) (DWP, 2001, p 114). Initiatives have also focused on healthcare delivery and specifically the NSF for older people (Recommendation 29). Concessionary fares for older people have been introduced in most local authorities. The fuel poverty strategy (Recommendation 12.1) has also benefited older people. However, overall, older people appear to be a relatively lower priority compared with other groups.

Ethnicity: Recommendations 31-33

31. Needs of minority ethnic groups
32. Services sensitive to needs of minority ethnic people and their health risks
33. Needs recognised in resource allocation, planning and provision

This area has been difficult to decipher, since few policies have been specifically aimed at minority ethnic groups. Examples do, however, address housing, employment, cancer services (including smoking cessation) and cover services provision and target setting (DWP, 2002a, p 124).

Gender: Recommendations 34-36

34. Accidents and suicides in young men
35. Psychosocial ill-health in young women
36. Disability in older women

The recommendations relating to gender are largely covered by others in the Inquiry (for example Recommendations 22, 35, and 36).

NHS: Recommendations 37-39

37. Access to effective care in relation to need
38. Allocation of NHS resources
39. Equity profile for local populations

The NHS's role in tackling health inequalities has been emphasised by *The NHS Plan* (DoH, 2000), *Shifting the balance of power* (DoH, 2001c) and the Wanless Report (Wanless, 2002). The government recognises that policy objectives for tackling health inequalities cannot be met by the NHS alone. An objective has been to maximise the NHS contribution, mainly through influencing 'mainstream' services. Particular initiatives have involved the 'realignment' of HAZs with their local health systems, "which will increase the capacity of PCTs to tackle health inequality issues" (DWP, 2002a, p 116). Also, HLCs are "expected to influence the wider determinants of health ... that can contribute to inequalities in health" (DWP, 2002a, p 115). Addressing the 'postcode lottery' (through NICE) will minimise geographical inequalities in access (Recommendation 37); NSFs will also contribute (Recommendation 37.3). The performance management of policies to tackle health inequalities is considered a priority and national targets will assist in this (Recommendation 37.4). However, ascertaining the role of the NHS per se in reducing health inequalities is problematic. The work of ACRA has generated "a total of £148m shared between 54 HAs" (for 2002-03) to recognise the additional effect that health inequalities have on the NHS (DoH, 2002c, p 2) (Recommendation 38). This shift in the formula is significant (especially as the years of life lost index has been "extended to included infant deaths under one year for all causes" (DoH, 2002c), the reduction of which is a DoH PSA target), but represents a relatively small proportion of total funding across increasingly large geographical areas (that comprise HAs). The Secretary of State indicated the future policy

direction in an answer to a Parliamentary Question (29 October 2002):

The existing formula used to allocate NHS resources is under review. Later this year [2002], when I announce resources for local health services, distribution will take place based on a new formula that takes better account of health needs, which I hope will contribute to reductions in health inequalities. (col 665)

The role of private practice has not been reviewed (Recommendation 38.4). The New guidance has been issued for DPH in relation to the publication of equity profiles of their district – a move welcomed by the Health Select Committee (Recommendation 39). Following publication of *Shifting the balance of power* (DoH, 2001c) (and its related reports), DPH have been appointed in each PCT; every StHA comprises a senior public health doctor/medical director and regional DPH have been appointed in the nine government offices of the regions. Although networks will coordinate activities at various levels, the role of public health in the transition to government offices of the regions, StHAs and PCTs remains uncertain.

3

Policy case study: tax and benefit reform

Introduction

Living standards and income are widely thought to have an effect on health and health inequalities, although the relationship is "not clearly understood" (Benzeval et al, 2000, p 376). Recent tax and benefit reforms are expected to have an impact on health inequalities, although the redistributive effects are only beginning to emerge.

The Independent Inquiry recognised the relationship between living standards and health inequalities. It recommended:

> Policies which will further reduce income inequalities and improve the living standards of households in receipt of social security benefits. (Recommendation 3)

This recommendation was considered to be "crucial" in tackling health inequalities.

The government has emphasised the need to address the causes of poverty rather than alleviating the symptoms. Current policy comprises three elements:

- promoting paid work;
- providing extra support to families and children;
- tackling child poverty.

Since 1997, the government has pursued these goals by means of:

- a partial integration of the tax and benefit systems;
- some income redistribution to poorer groups, notably families with children;
- tax credits;

- minima (such as the minimum income guarantee for pensioners and national minimum wage) – minima do not necessarily address inequality across the social gradient; rather they provide a 'floor'.

Here, income distribution and life span distribution show how tax and benefit reforms are seeking to improve living standards and reduce inequalities.

Income distribution and redistribution

Problem

The Inquiry noted the studies that demonstrated an association between poor health and material disadvantage, such as between all-cause mortality and the Townsend deprivation score. However, the Inquiry warned that "available evidence is insufficient to confirm or deny a causal relationship between changes in income distribution and the parallel deterioration in inequalities in some areas of ill-health" (p 33). This warning affects policy formulation, since "much of the available evidence on the relationship between income and health is of little help in forming policies to reduce health inequalities" (Benzeval et al, 2000, p 375).

The features of income and its distribution in the UK are stark. As earnings are the largest component of income, growth in wages plays a large part in the changes in inequality. For example, households with more than one adult but all unemployed (workless households) rose from 8% to 17% between 1979 and 1999 (Brewer and Gregg, 2001). Moreover, half of those in the poorest group in 1991 were still there in 1996 (HM Treasury, 1999, p 7).

Policy

The government has rejected the 'standard method' of redistribution through the tax and benefit system alone, and other methods have been sought to enhance the opportunities related to education, training and paid employment. While the government initially accepted the financial framework that they had inherited in 1997, some redistribution has since taken place through tax credits, tax thresholds and benefit levels. The 1998 and 1999 Budgets were mildly redistributive, weighted towards the poorest families. The IFS (2000, 2002) assessed the distributional impact of major fiscal reform since 1997 (Figures 3.1 and 3.2), which shows the significant distributional changes since 1997, especially in the 2002 Budget and the emphasis placed on children.

Direct and indirect taxation

The Inquiry noted that a "fairer tax system" would raise the income of poor people who are employed and minimise the "poverty trap" for those able to work. It notes that the shift towards indirect taxation in the last two decades, and favours a more progressive tax burden.

Taxation of spending/consumption helps explain the extent of inequality. Generally, direct taxes are progressive; for example:

> The proportion of gross income paid in direct tax by the top fifth of households is double that paid by the bottom fifth: 24% compared with 12%. Indirect taxes have the opposite effect to direct taxes. (ONS, 2000, p 45)

The regressive nature of indirect taxes is shown in Table 3.1; there have been no significant changes to indirect taxation recently.

The impact of taxation can be gauged from changes in the Gini coefficient – a measure which rates the degree of inequality (with lower

Table 3.1: Indirect taxation in terms of disposable income and expenditure for non-retired households, 1998–99 (%)

	Bottom quintile	Top quintile	All non-retired households
As % of disposable income	33.5	15.4	20.8
As % of household expenditure	21.8	16.2	18.9

Source: ONS (2000, Table G)

Figure 3.1: The impact of fiscal measures by decile, 1997–2001 and 1997–2002

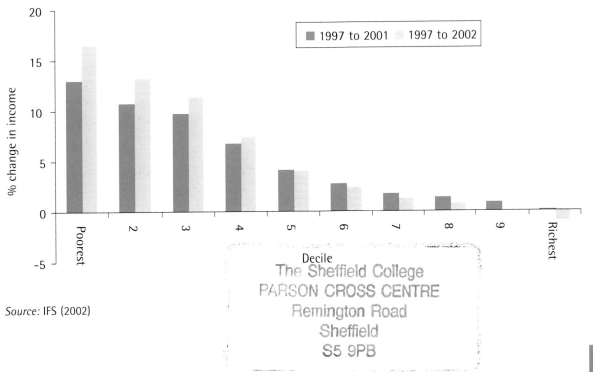

Source: IFS (2002)

Figure 3.2: Distributional impact of major fiscal reforms announced since July 1997, by family type

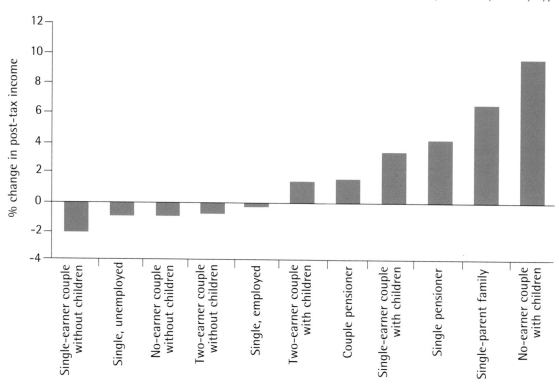

scores equating with a more even distribution). Table 3.2 shows the moderating effect of different forms of taxation – cash benefits have a more redistributive effect than taxation; direct tax reduces the coefficient while indirect taxes raise it.

A significant change in policy took place in the 2002 Budget by the government "openly affirming the role for redistributive taxation in creating a fairer and more inclusive society" (Catalyst Trust, 2002, Figure 3.1). This strategy

may be undermined by what some have considered as an insufficient 'safety net', an 'over-reliance' on means-tested benefits, a 'coercive' element in welfare-to-work and wider socioeconomic influences.

Life-span distribution

The government's policies indicate a "good understanding of the life-course influences" on health inequalities (Benzeval et al, 2000, p 391). Across government, the emphasis has been on families with children and on paid employment (although the poorest groups are households in which no one has paid employment). This is in line with the Inquiry's recommendations and should, in due course, help to tackle the intergenerational transmission of poverty.

In short, groups who have an above average risk of low income (in 2002) are found across the life span, including workless households, families with children, pensioners, minority ethnic groups, disabled people, local authority or housing association tenants, people with no educational qualifications, and people who live in the North East of England or in London (ONS, 2002).

Table 3.2: Gini coefficient, 1998-99 (% shares of equivalised income)

	Gini coefficient
Original income plus cash benefits	53 (%)
Gross income minus direct taxes	38 (%)
Disposable income minus indirect taxes	35 (%)
Post-tax income plus benefits in kind (education, health and so on)	39 (%)
Final income	

Source: ONS (2000, Chart 1 and Table A)

Children

Problem

The Inquiry recognised that:

A child, and additional children, has a much greater impact on the standard of living of poorer than better-off households. Yet current levels of benefits are not generous ... relative to average incomes. (p 34)

It also reported that benefit levels were insufficient to meet the "minimum needs of children" (p 34).

In the last 20 years, the incidence of childhood poverty has doubled (ONS, 2002), making children the poorest group in the UK (replacing pensioners). The UK has one of the highest rates of child poverty in OECD countries, with one fifth of children living in workless households in 1996 compared with an EU average of 11% (Brewer and Gregg, 2001, p 4; see also DWP, 2002a). The rise of childhood poverty has been associated with increased earnings inequality, the rise of lone parent households, and the increasing proportion of households with children and no working adult.

By 2001, there were 2.7 million children living in households with below 60% of median household income (on a before housing costs basis; this figure rises to 3.9 million children after housing costs) (ONS, 2002). These figures equate with a drop in the number of children in poverty on this measure of around ½ million children since 1996/7 (ONS, 2002).

The consequences of child poverty are evident in children's subsequent earnings, their educational attainment, poorer adult health and the transmission of poverty through worklessness, even after controlling for child ability and aspects of family background (Brewer and Gregg, 2001, p 6).

Policy

In 1999 the government announced a target of ending child poverty within a generation. The *2002 Spending Review* reaffirmed the government's commitment to tackle child poverty by:

Reducing the number of children living in low-income households by at least a quarter by 2004 as a contribution towards the broader target of halving child poverty by 2010 and eradicating it by 2020. (DWP PSA, 2002, see Appendix D, page 67)

Poverty is commonly defined as poor households with incomes at less than 60% of the national median income. In 2002, the DWP sought to clarify this definition by consulting on four possible new measures of child poverty:

- a small number of multidimensional headline indicators;
- constructing an index from headline indicators;
- a headline measure of consistent poverty;
- a core set of indicators (DWP, 2002b).

This exercise was designed to overcome concerns that, at the moment, the strategy appears clearer than the target (Brewer and Gregg, 2001, p 27).

The policies to meet the objective have been based on four elements (DWP, 2001).

Direct financial support:

- Children's Tax Credit (supporting low income families with children);
- Childcare Tax Credit (helping to pay for childcare);
- Integrated Child Credit (combining all income-related benefits and tax credit support from 2003);
- Working Families' Tax Credit (supporting families on low and moderate incomes);
- increases in Child Benefit and child allowances in Income Support;
- personal tax and benefit reforms (such as changes to Incapacity Benefit and maternity/paternity provision).

Workless households:

- New Deal for Lone Parents (offering a programme of job-search, training, childcare and in-work benefit information);
- National Childcare Strategy (including out-of-school clubs);
- Childcare Tax Credit (supporting low-income families to pay for childcare).

Long-term consequences of poverty:

- Sure Start programmes (focusing on services for 0- to 4-year-olds);
- Sure Start Maternity Grant (paid to recipients of Income Support and other benefits);
- Children's Fund (providing £450 million (2001-04) for 5- to 13-year-old children);
- Connexions service (bridging the education–work gap for 13- to 19-year-olds).

Early years interventions:

- targets for numeracy and literacy in primary school education;
- provision of free early education places (to all 4-year-olds) and its extension to 3-year-olds (by September 2004);
- creation of the Children and Young People's Unit (to coordinate investment in services);
- Sure Start programme (see Chapter 5);
- Early Excellence Centres (offering integrated early years services in 35 centres);
- Foundation Stage (setting Early Learning Goals for children in the reception year);
- targets to reduce truancy and school exclusions (by a third by 2002, and truancy rates by a further 10% by 2004);
- Education Action Zones;
- Excellence in Cities initiative;
- Special Educational Needs Coordinators (supporting early years education).

Following the *2002 Spending Review*, Sure Start, childcare and early years programmes were brought together in a single interdepartmental unit.

Progress

These initiatives have provided a reasonably coherent framework, although progress to date has been inconclusive. The redistributive effect of various policies is illustrated by Figure 3.3.

Evidence indicates that from 1996/7 to 2000/01 "there was a fall of 1.3 million in the number of children below 60% of the 1996/7 median income held constant in real terms on a before housing cost basis" (ONS, 2002; see also DWP, 2002a, p 60). Some evidence has suggested that infant mortality rates in the "worst and best health areas" have started to reduce (Shaw et al,

2001). It is unclear whether, or how far, these changes are attributable to policy interventions per se. For example, the WFTC generated over one million claims in its first year. Also, there has been a reduction in the number of children in workless households from 17.3% to 15.8% between 1999 and 2000 (Brewer and Gregg, 2001, p 22). The DWP suggests that progress in reducing the number of children living in low-income households (by 300,000 children to 2000/01, after housing costs) is in line with the PSA target of reducing such numbers by a quarter by 2002 (from 1998/99) (DWP, 2002a, p 61).

However, despite evidence of some redistribution, children who are lifted out of poverty still tend to be the closest to the poverty level: policies may only marginally improve the situation for the poorest children. Also, one sixth of children still live in persistent poverty (between 1997 and 2000) (DWP, 2002a, p 61). Policies must therefore be sustained, extended or accelerated to prevent these children falling back into poverty and to reach other children who remain in poverty (CASE, 2000; Catalyst Trust, 2002). The Integrated Child Credit (to be introduced from April 2003) will provide further support for reducing child poverty as well as combining and simplifying existing benefits. However, the immediate impact of ICC is expected to be small (Brewer et al, 2001).

Working-age adults

Problem

The Inquiry reported that nearly 25% of households contain at least one person who receives Income Support (p 32). Noting the association of increasingly poor health with increasing material disadvantage, the Inquiry favoured a "shift of resources to the less well-off both in and out of work" (p 33).

Poverty among working-age adults is revealed by recent ONS figures:

In 2000/1, on a Before Housing Cost basis, there were 4.9 million working-age adults living in households with below 60% of median household income. (ONS, 2002)

Figure 3.3: Financial impact for families as a result of children's measures introduced by 2003

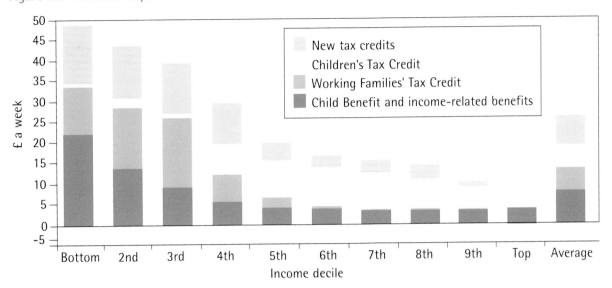

Legend:
- New tax credits
- Children's Tax Credit
- Working Families' Tax Credit
- Child Benefit and income-related benefits

Y-axis: £ a week
X-axis: Income decile — Bottom, 2nd, 3rd, 4th, 5th, 6th, 7th, 8th, 9th, Top, Average

Source: DWP (2002a, p 48)

This equates to 6.6 million adults after housing costs – a figure that has changed little between 1994/95 and 2000/01.

Poverty is also related to workless households, earnings inequality and earnings immobility:

> More than half the people below retirement age who are living on low incomes live in households where no one has a job. (HM Treasury, 1999, p 7)

Also, job loss has profound consequences associated with lower rates of pay in a new job compared with the previous job. The gap between pre-unemployment wages and wages 2-3 years after unemployment has risen from 11% (1982-86) to 20% (1992-97) for men (Brewer and Gregg, 2001, p 3).

Policy

Paid employment is promoted as the best way to avoid poverty and social exclusion; work is both prevention and cure (DWP, 2001, p 74).

> At the centre of our strategy is the belief that, for most families, work is the best route out of poverty. (DWP, 2002b, p 11)

Policy therefore seeks to overcome the barriers to employment.

Policies supporting working-age adults:

- New Deal for Young People (programme for those unemployed and claiming Jobseeker's Allowance for over six months);
- New Deal 25 Plus (involving a mandatory programme for long-term unemployed people);
- New Deal for Disabled People (programme to help disabled people who want to work);
- New Deal for Partners (providing advice, support and guidance for non-working partners who are receiving working-age benefits);
- New Deal 50 Plus (involving a voluntary programme for economically inactive older people);
- Working Families' Tax Credit (WFTC; providing financial support to low-income householders who are employed);
- Disabled Person's Tax Credit;
- Employment Tax Credit (extending WFTC to low-income families, from 2003);
- National Childcare Strategy (which has generated over 380,000 places since 1997; DWP, 2001, p 31);
- changes to the tax and benefit system;
- increased child allowances in Income Support;
- Sure Start maternity grant;
- benefit level changes (such as Child Benefit);
- tax threshold changes (such as lower earnings limit);
- national minimum wage (in conjunction with WFTC, providing a guaranteed minimum

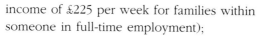

income of £225 per week for families within someone in full-time employment);

- Action Teams for Jobs (offering coordinated programmes to get long-term unemployed people back to work);
- Connexions (bridging the education–work gap);
- Jobcentre Plus (linking benefit and employment services).

Progress

The promotion of paid work is not simply a question of financial resources, because it must also be accompanied by childcare, transport and family-friendly employment policies. This has been recognised and there is some evidence that strategies across these areas are beginning to have a positive effect. The ONS (2002) claims that between 1996/97 and 2000/01, "there was a fall of 1.2 million in the number of working-age adults below 60% of the 1996/7 median income, before housing costs". However, the number of working-age people living in households with a relatively low income has remained 'broadly constant' at 15% (before housing costs; 20% after housing costs) between 1996/97 and 2000/01. (The figures for absolute low income fell by four percentage points over the same period.) Similarly, in three out of four years (1997-2000) 7% of working-age people were living in low-income households (DWP, 2002a, p 66).

Among specific groups, there are some signs of progress. The greatest impact of the NMW has been among women, who account for about 70% of the 1.5 million workers who benefit (DWP, 2001, p 84). Also, up to June 2001, 670,000 people joined the New Deal for Young People, of whom nearly half moved into employment (DWP, 2001, p 76). Improvements in employment rates are mirrored in other groups (DWP, 2002a):

- older workers: from 64.7% in 1997 to 68.1% in 2002;
- minority ethnic groups: from 57.3% in 1997 to 58.3% in 2002;
- lone parents: from 45.6% in 1997 to 53.6% in 2002;
- disabled people: from 43.5% in 1998 to 48.0% in 2002.

(The employment rate of lone parents has been incorporated as a PSA target; DWP, 2002a.) The DWP (2002a) indicates that these data provide positive trends since the baseline, but the rates for minority ethnic groups and older people are not "moving in the right direction" (p 2). As these increases have generally been larger than the overall employment rate, the 'employment rate gap' (between these groups and the working-age population) has been reduced.

Mothers seeking work still face barriers in terms of childcare, partly because of the array of providers and their variable cost and quality. There also remains a shortfall in provision (Paull et al, 2002). Policies such as the WFTC and other credits may surprisingly appear to have had a limited impact on the choices of mothers. The "generous childcare subsidies under the WFTC are predicted to have relatively limited effect on employment, raising the employment rate for single mothers by 3% points" (Paull et al, 2002). Paull et al conclude that "childcare subsidies may have high costs for the government with little impact on mothers' employment".

Older people

Problem

Until recently, pensioners were the poorest group across the life span. Although children now occupy this position, pensioner poverty is still widespread: in 2000/01, two million pensioners were living below 60% of the 1996/97 median income (before housing costs). Although this represents a fall of 500,000 since 1996/97 (ONS, 2002), one in four pensioners still lives in a low-income household (after housing costs) (DWP, 2002a).

Policy

Most policies have focused on families with children but there are several policies that have targeted older people, including:

- minimum income guarantee;
- winter fuel payments (as part of the Fuel Poverty Strategy);
- Pension Credit (from 2003);
- concessionary fares (see Chapter 6);
- above-inflation increases to the basic state pension.

Policies were maintained or extended in the pre-Budget statement (in November 2001):

- guaranteeing a minimum increase of £100 per annum to the basic state pension for single pensioners and £160 for couples in 2003-04;
- maintaining winter fuel payments paid to eight million households at £200 per annum for rest of this Parliament (HM Treasury, 2001a).

Progress

The DWP (2002c) found that, from 1994/95 to 2000/01, there had been "little consistent change in the percentage of pensioners living in low-income households" (p 5). One in four of the two million older people live in poverty (after housing costs), and single female pensioners are at most risk of poverty. Moreover, 17% of older people lived in low-income households in three of the four years between 1997 and 2000. However, the DWP's (2002a) assessment of progress reports that absolute low income among older people has fallen from 27% in 1996/97 to 15% in 2000/01 (p 73).

The redistributive impact of taxation and benefits on retired households is shown in Table 3.3, which indicates that the ratio of the lowest quintile and the highest quintile is reduced from 1:18 to 1:2.8. The effect is also demonstrated by changes to the Gini coefficient (Table 3.4).

Table 3.4: Gini coefficients for retired households, 1998–99

	Gini coefficient
Original income	66
Gross income	30
Disposable	28
Post-tax income	31

Source: ONS (2001, Table J)

Overall assessment across the life span

By understanding the factors which influence people's trajectories through life, it is possible to develop strategies to reduce the incidence, direction and severity of events which place people at greater risk of disadvantage. (HM Treasury, 1999, p 5, para 1.05)

Recognition of the need to tackle poverty across the life span is in line with the Inquiry's recommendations and is evident across government. This is most clearly demonstrated in the *2002 Cross-cutting Review* on health inequalities (HM Treasury/DoH, 2002), which used a life-course approach in its analysis of the interventions needed and "identified the early years of childhood and older age as life stages where action to tackle health inequalities is particularly important" (HM Treasury/DoH, 2002, p 8, para 22).

Policies have so far focused predominantly on families with children, with less help going to older people. Workless households with children have gained most (Table 3.5).

Table 3.3: The effects of taxes and benefits on retired households by lowest and highest quintile groups, 1998–99 (£ per annum)

	Bottom quintile	Top quintile
Original income	1,020	18,540
Final income	6,790	19,270

Source: ONS (2001, Table K)

Table 3.5: Distributional impact by family type of fiscal reform since 1997

	Change (%)
No earner with children	+10
Single parent	+6
Single pensioner	+4
Single-earner couple with children	+3
Single-earner couple with no children	−2

Source: Benzeval et al (2000)

However, given the deep-seated nature of poverty, policies have yet to translate fully into observable reductions. Thus, the DWP (2002c) concluded that:

from 1994/5 to 2000/1, the percentage of the population living in low income households, as defined by contemporary mean or median, showed no large or consistent change. (p 25)

This illustrates the challenges that remain.

Conclusions

The government has:

• signalled that paid employment and fiscal redistribution are the crucial means of tackling poverty;
• introduced policies that focus on routes into employment;
• adopted a life-span perspective by emphasising children and families (especially those out of work) relative to the needs of older people.

These approaches are in line with the Inquiry's recommendations and represent a positive start. More remains to be done, however.

Since many policies have only recently been implemented and some have yet to be introduced, it is too early to judge their overall effectiveness. Also, the wider socioeconomic context (notably income inequalities) may undermine the positive effects of policy. Evidence about the link between income and health inequalities is equivocal but, if they are positively associated, the rapid wage growth of recent years may hamper these policies. Rising tax revenues have enabled redistribution to poorer social groups. The interactive effect of redistributive policies and other social programmes is also unknown. At this stage, therefore, it remains unclear whether tax and benefit policies are sufficient in themselves, whether they are sustainable in the long term, and whether cross-departmental support can be maintained.

While policy developments are encouraging and should be sustained, it is essential that the Treasury and the DWP continue to pursue tax and benefit policies that are conducive to tackling (health) inequalities. While the government recognises the importance of fiscal policy, tax and welfare benefits in this context, it is unfortunate that these are outside the remit of the *Cross-cutting Review*. They are essential components of any strategy to tackle health inequalities and it is not sufficient for the strategy to 'sit alongside' policies in those areas (HM Treasury/DoH, 2002). There is a need, therefore, for closer dialogue with service departments about the type of tax and benefit changes that would be supportive of policies in other areas. This dialogue would be aided by the inclusion of tax and benefit policy within the remit of the DA(SER), which is to oversee the delivery of the strategy on health inequalities.

In summary, the impacts of tax and benefit reforms are emerging but the effects on health inequalities are not yet evident and may not be for several years. The policies being pursued are appropriate but need to be sustained and even extended over a substantial period of time if they are to have any impact on health inequalities. Changes in poverty levels also need to be accompanied by changes resulting from other policies to tackle health inequalities (such as smoking cessation, housing conditions and educational attainment). Tax and benefit reforms need to be included within the remit of intergovernmental arrangements for joining up efforts to tackle health inequalities and to be an integral part of the strategy.

4

Policy case study: performance management

Introduction

Setting targets and measuring achievements are crucial tasks in ensuring that objectives are met across government. Analysis of these systems explains how and why progress in tackling health inequalities might be made and sustained. Performance management is currently the prime mechanism to effect change (NAO, 2001a).

Performance management is a "set of managerial instruments designed to secure optimal performance ... over time, in line with policy objectives" (Smith, 2002, p 105). It involves:

- *Guidance:* transmission of policy objectives;
- *Monitoring:* information regarding achievement of objectives;
- *Response:* remedial action (if required) and promotion of continuous improvement (Smith, 2002).

Performance management is problematic when short-term managerial objectives need to be balanced against longer-term strategic goals, and when performance may be difficult to measure and attribute.

The Independent Inquiry made recommendations relating to performance management in the NHS.

37.   Providing equitable access to effective care in relation to need should be a governing principle of all policies in the NHS. Priority should be given to the achievement of equity in planning, implementation and delivery of services at every level of the NHS.

37.4.   We recommend that performance management in relation to the national performance management framework is focused on achieving more equitable access, provision and targeting of effective services in relation to need in both primary and hospital sectors.

37.5.   We recommend that the Department of Health and NHS Executive set out their responsibilities for furthering the principle of equity of access to effective health and social care, and that health authorities, working with Primary Care Groups and providers on local clinical governance, agree priorities and objectives for reducing inequities in access to effective care.

This chapter examines public service agreements (PSAs) as an example of a cross-governmental approach to performance management. Later, it addresses performance management in the DoH and DfES, because of their pivotal role in current policy to tackle health inequalities and because they face contrasting pressures from within their departments relating to mainstream services.

Targets for health inequalities: the role of public service agreements

The performance of departments is assessed by various measures. The key measures are PSAs, which were first introduced in 1998. They are 'contracts' between the Treasury and the department, acting as high level measurable targets. PSAs "bring together in a single document important information on the aim, objectives and performance targets for each of the main departments in Government" (HM Treasury, 2000, p 3). Each PSA contains service delivery agreements (SDAs), which provide "more detailed outputs which departments will need to focus on to achieve their objectives" (p 2). The Secretary of State in each department is normally responsible for the achievement of PSAs. Most departments have PSAs that are relevant to tackling health inequalities (see Appendix D).

Over time, PSAs have been reduced in number and changed in scope. PSA targets were reduced from about 30 to about 10 per department in 2000 (Gray and Jenkins, 2001, p 210); these amounted to "around 130" in the PSAs published in the *2002 Spending Review*. Also,

> The percentage of PSA targets that address outcomes increased from 15% in 1999-2002 to 68% for 2001-2004. (NAO, 2001a, para 3)

The emphasis on outcomes is unusual compared with other countries (NAO, 2001a) – a development welcomed by the Treasury Select Committee. PSA targets now also focus more on the link between spending and performance; this link was developed further in the PSAs published in the *2002 Spending Review*.

The extent to which PSAs represent 'joined-up' activity has been questioned. Attention has focused on the balance between collaboration with other departments and a vertical 'silo' approach. The Treasury Select Committee welcomed the cross-cutting PSAs but emphasised the need for clear accountability. It noted, for example, the support for Sure Start PSA and a "clear designation of the responsible Minister, the creation of a unit with a specified head, a separate vote (estimate) for its expenditure and an additional accounting officer" (para 30). However, the Secretary of State for Education and Employment was responsible at Cabinet level and the Minister for Public Health held day-to-day responsibility for the unit. The Sure Start PSA was extended in 2002 to include 'childcare and early years' – the Ministerial responsibility for which had yet to be determined. The four targets for the 2002 PSA were similar to the 2000 targets; revisions included the addition, removal or adjustment of percentage changes for targets.

Performance management of health inequalities in the Department of Health

Targets for health inequalities

The Independent Inquiry did not recommend targets for tackling health inequalities as they were considered beyond the remit of the Inquiry (Marmot, 1999). The Green Paper *Our healthier nation* (DoH, 1998b) also rejected them. It did not:

> propose *at this stage* to set national targets to narrow health inequalities between social classes, different parts of the country, ethnic groups, and men and women.... Because the causation is so complex and many factors inter-react, it is not possible to set realistic quantified targets for greater equality *at this stage*. (Exworthy and Powell, 2000, pp 55-6 emphasis added)

However, *The NHS Plan* (DoH, 2000) stated that health inequality targets would be set; these were published in February 2001.

> Starting with children under one year, by 2010, to reduce by at least 10% the gap in mortality between manual groups and the population as a whole.

> Starting with health authorities, by 2010, to reduce by at least 10% the gap between the fifth of areas with the lowest life expectancy at birth and the population as a whole.

These targets were combined in a DoH PSA in July 2002:

> By 2010, reduce inequalities in health outcomes by 10% as measured by infant mortality and life expectancy at birth. (DoH, 2002, see Appendix D, page 65)

This builds on earlier target-setting processes and will need to be translated into the performance management systems of the DoH and of local agencies. They address socioeconomic and geographical inequalities, across the life span. Although they focus only on mortality, they "underpin a much wider range of initiatives addressing, for example, morbidity, disability and social care" (DWP, 2001, p 55). The targets are under review following the abolition of health authorities and revisions to social class classifications. In March 2002, the DoH 'updated' progress on these targets.

Infant mortality

The DoH (2001d) noted 'little change' in the gap between the infant mortality rate (IMR) among manual social classes and the general population; the gap showed a 'slight widening', by 0.5% between 1997-99 and 1998-2000. However, by 2006, the IMR is expected to drop from 5.7 deaths per thousand live births to below 5.0 (CPAG, 2001).

Life expectancy

The DoH (2002a) noted that "the gap between the 'best' (Kensington, Chelsea and Westminster) and 'worst' (Manchester) widened to 7.7 years for men and 6.6 years for women". Further, in the 'worst' fifth of health authorities, life expectancy is 2.2 years lower for men and 1.7 years lower for women (CPAG, 2001). However, ONS (2002) figures show that the gap in life expectancy between social classes I and V has narrowed from 9 years to 7 years (1997-99). If the gap had begun to narrow by 1999 (that is, before many of the policies designed to do so had taken their full effect), this augurs well for further reductions.

The DoH has announced other targets that support strategies to tackle health inequalities (see Appendix D); teenage pregnancy and smoking are illustrated here.

Teenage pregnancy

Targets: "By achieving agreed local conception reduction targets, to reduce the national under 18 conception rate by 15% by 2004, and 50% by 2010 while reducing the gap in rates between the worst fifth of [electoral] wards and the average by at least a quarter" (DoH, 2002b, p 7).

Progress: "The under-18 and under-16 conception rates both fell by more than 6 per cent during the first two years of the implementation of the strategy" (DWP, 2002a, p 88).

Smoking

Targets: "To reduce smoking rates among manual groups from 32% to 26% by 2010"; "By 2010, reduce cancer mortality rates by more than 20% in people under 75 by 2010, aiming to improve the health of the worst off in particular" (DoH, 2002b, p 7).

Progress: "In 2000, the proportion of women who smoked during pregnancy was 19%". Smoking rates still exhibit a strong socioeconomic gradient: 31% of adults in manual groups, 23% in non-manual groups. Although the gap has narrowed to 9 percentage points in 2000 (from 11 percentage points in 1998), smoking rates in non-manual groups have edged upwards since the mid-1990s. (All figures from DWP, 2002a, p 113.)

For some targets, there is some evidence of progress but generally there is insufficient data or insufficient time has elapsed to enable robust conclusions to be made about policy interventions.

'Consultation on a plan for delivery'

In 2001, the DoH (2001b) published a consultation document on future strategies for tackling health inequalities (in England), seeking opinions on a 'basket' of indicators to support the two national targets, on the role of PCTs and on the further actions at national and local levels.

The consultation document proposed a framework for different levels of indicators:

- national targets;
- high level indicators;
- national/regional basket of indicators (including a broader set from which regions can choose their priorities);
- local basket of indicators (from which local partnerships can choose).

These indicators could apply to local performance management systems such as:

- local strategic partnerships;
- health improvement and modernisation programmes and community strategies;
- local PSAs;
- performance of key initiatives (such as HAZ, Sure Start and New Deal);

- NHS performance assessment framework;
- Best Value performance indicators.

The results of the consultation were published in June 2002. They noted respondents' support for the basket of indicators but the need to integrate them with indicators used by other departments was also stressed. Respondents favoured a wider range of indicators and suggested 'possible areas that might be included':

- measures of quality of life;
- social capital;
- environmental health;
- rural and urban communities;
- older people;
- mental health;
- access to food;
- stroke, chronic pulmonary disease, diabetes;
- oral health (DoH, 2002b, p 25).

Local performance management

The public health Green Paper *Our healthier nation* (DoH, 1998b) encouraged local health inequality targets. Their development involves the integration of health inequalities strategies into mainstream planning, which may be achieved via the inclusion within performance management systems. *The NHS Plan* (DoH, 2000) proposed a new system for performance management based on 'earned autonomy' (according to 'traffic light' status) and a Modernisation Agency. The 'traffic light' status assigned to organisations will be based on delivery of national targets and overall performance as measured against the performance assessment framework. The approach involves measurement against the delivery of minimum requirements (the 'must-dos') and against organisational performance.

The DoH claimed that:

> The government is committed to tackling health inequalities and believes that the traffic lighting system will be an important instrument in raising standards nationally to a uniformly acceptable level. (2001e, p 3)

As different organisations and areas start from different positions, the DoH recognised that performance measures needed to include a value added element, to reward performance over time and to reflect absolute standards. The DoH has also recognised the greater needs of some areas by providing additional funding to reflect local health inequality.

In addition, the DoH's (2002d) priorities and planning framework included a central role for health inequalities. It states the priorities for health and social care:

- *improving access to all services* through better emergency care, reduced waiting, increased booking for appointments and admission and more choice for patients;
- *focusing on improving services and outcomes* in cancer, coronary heart disease, mental health, older people, improving life chances for children, improving overall experience of patients, reducing health inequalities, contributing to the cross-government drive to reduce drug misuse. (para 3.2)

Particular emphasis is placed on "making measurable progress", "developing capacity" and "changing the way the whole system works" (para 1.3). To this end, lead agencies will be responsible for ensuring the process of developing elements of local delivery plans (covering a StHA but based on PCT level plans). This document stresses the need for a more stable planning framework of three years. Although health inequality programmes contain longer-term objectives, it is important that the planning framework is also congruent with the performance management of health inequality programmes.

The performance of NHS organisations is assessed using the performance assessment framework, which involves six dimensions.

The DoH published national figures and performance by health authority. However, the health authority (as a unit of analysis) may mask local inequalities by, for example, covering large areas and containing diverse populations (targets are being reviewed following the authorities' abolition and the creation of StHAs). Tables 4.2 to 4.5 illustrate the progress made relating to health improvement (as examples of the performance assessment framework). Few dimensions specifically refer to inequalities but they do overcome criticisms of narrow performance indicators (such as finished consultant episodes or efficiency index). Indicators of progress in tackling health

Table 4.1: NHS performance assessment framework and possible local strategies

Dimensions of performance	Examples of indicators	Examples of action on inequalities
Health improvement	Life expectancy	Reducing health inequalities through economic, social and environmental action within and beyond the NHS.
Fair access	Infant mortality rate Breast screening	Identifying potential inequalities as a result of geography, socioeconomic group, ethnicity, sex and age. (The number of 'heart operations' in areas with low rates of operations despite high rates of CHD are being increased; DWP, 2002a, p 112.)
Effective delivery	Surgical rates for coronary heart disease Childhood immunisations	Addressing inequalities that result from care/services, which are inappropriate for a particular group or community.
Efficiency	Primary care management of chronic conditions Day case rate	Reducing inappropriate use of emergency services or non-attendance by individuals and groups experiencing access problems.
Patient/carer experience	Length of stay Six month in-patient waiting	Reducing inequalities created by services that are not people-centred.
Health outcome	Access to a GP Emergency admission for children with lower respiratory infection	Identifying those users of services who need additional social support to rehabilitate following NHS care.
	Smokers continuing to quit (after four weeks)	

Source: Bull and Hamer (2001)

inequalities need to include structure, process and outcome components so that strategies can be monitored in the short term to long term.

A performance fund, established by the Modernisation Agency, will aid local improvements. All NHS trusts will share this fund, but 'best' performing agencies will be free to use their share for any "performance improvement purpose". The Modernisation Agency will direct the funds of the 'worst' agencies. The fund will amount to roughly 2% of agencies' budgets by 2003 (Smith, 2002, p 108).

Following the publication of *Shifting the balance of power* (DoH, 2001c), PCTs are the local agencies which will:

- commission acute services;
- develop primary care services;
- improve the population's health.

The third objective involves health needs assessment, preparation of plans to reduce health inequalities and collaboration in local strategic partnerships (LSPs) (HDA, 2002). However, it might be eclipsed by the immediacy of the first two objectives (Exworthy et al, 2002); hence, its role needs to be emphasised. For example, the inclusion of health inequalities within the remit of local authority scrutiny committees would strengthen local performance management systems across interagency boundaries.

Table 4.2: Health improvement: national performance

	Previous year data	Current year data	National % improvement
Life expectancy, males	74.7	75.2	0.7
Life expectancy, females	79.8	80.1	0.4
Deaths from cancer	133.4	130.6	2.1
Deaths from circulatory diseases	127.0	120.4	5.2
Suicide rates	9.3	9.4	−1.0
Deaths from accidents	16.4	16.3	0.7
Conceptions below 18	46.5	44.7	4.1
Decayed, missing or filled teeth from five-year-old children	1.5	1.4	2.4
Infant mortality rate	5.9	5.7	3.4

Notes:

Deaths from cancer: age-standardised mortality rate from all malignant neoplasms in people aged under 75, per 100,000.

Deaths from circulatory disease: age-standardised mortality rate from all circulatory diseases in persons aged under 75, per 100,000.

Suicide rates: age-standardised mortality rate from suicide and injury undetermined whether accidentally or purposely inflicted, per 100,000.

Deaths from accidents: age-standardised mortality rate from accidents, per 100,000.

Conceptions under 18: number of conceptions among girls aged under 18 resident in an area per 1,000 girls aged 15-17 years.

Teeth: average number of teeth per five-year-old child that are actively decayed, missing or filled.

Infant mortality rate: number of deaths in infants under one year per 1,000 live births.

Source: DoH (2002e)

Table 4.3: Life expectancy, males (selected health authorities) (1995-97 to 1997-99)

		Improvement	
	Years	(%)[a]	Band[b]
East London and City	72.6	+1.0	4
Kensington, Chelsea and Westminster	77.5	+1.1	5
Manchester	70.2	+0.1	1
Tees	73.6	+1.0	5

Notes: [a] Over various time periods. [b] 1=poor, 5=good.
Source: DoH (2002e)

Table 4.4: Life expectancy, females (selected health authorities) (1995-97 to 1997-99)

		Improvement	
	Years	(%)[a]	Band[b]
East London and City	79.2	+1.0%	5
Kensington, Chelsea and Westminster	82.4	+0.9%	5
Manchester	76.6	−0.4%	1
Tees	78.7	+0.3%	3

Notes: [a] Over various time periods. [b] 1=poor, 5=good.
Source: DoH (2002e)

Table 4.5: Infant mortality rate (selected health authorities) (1996-98 to 1997-99)

	Rate, per 1,000 live births	Improvement (%)[a]	Band[b]
East London and City	7.7	−1.3%	3
Kensington, Chelsea and Westminster	6.6	+10.8%	4
Manchester	8.2	−7.9%	2
Tees	5.2	+16.1%	5

Notes: [a] Over various time periods. [b] 1=poor, 5=good.
Source: DoH (2002e)

The DoH will measure progress on tackling health inequalities using the returns provided by the monitoring electronic service and financial framework (SAFF), the primary instrument for local planning. For 2001/02, of the 110 issues that were measured by the SAFF, eight were applicable to health inequality strategies:

- preparation of the infrastructure for changes to child health and antenatal screening programmes;
- contribution to the development of Sure Start and learn lessons from mainstream services;
- production of a joint health authority/local authority report on progress with teenage pregnancy strategy;
- increase in the number of GPs working in deprived areas;
- 600 severely disabled children to receive support services (disability register);
- produce a health youth offending team (YOT) action plan with social services departments;
- annual health assessment for every looked after child;
- review of the NHS contribution to YOTs with social services departments.

Policies to tackle health inequalities have been incorporated into performance management systems for DoH activity at national and, potentially at least, at local level. The PSA target for health inequalities is a significant development and other targets will also contribute. The performance management system for tackling health inequalities must closely relate to these and the forthcoming basket of indicators. The delivery plan should show how far this is likely to be achieved. However, more needs to be done to ensure that the impact of policies on health inequalities is assessed properly.

Performance management in the Department for Education and Skills

The Independent Inquiry stressed the role of educational qualifications in shaping an individual's labour market position and thus influencing income and housing. Education also equips individuals with practical, social and emotional knowledge, and aids their full participation in society. The importance of pre-school education in nurseries was also recognised by the Inquiry, because all forms of pre-school attendance have been shown to have a positive impact on tests taken at aged seven and on later school attendance.

School-based factors can raise educational attainment, which will have long-term benefits. However, since the performance of the weakest pupils has not risen, the gap between the top and bottom achievers has widened. The proportion of young people gaining no GCSEs, for example, has fallen since the late 1980s.

Policy: national objective and targets

The DfES has set objectives and targets for improving educational attainment; most accord with a focus on the wider determinants of health. The objectives and targets for two groups are given in Table 4.6 as examples of national policy.

Similar objectives and targets have been set by the DfES for its contribution to neighbourhood renewal strategies. DfES has also 'committed' itself to extending Sure Start by 2004, to delivering a national Connexions service by 2002/03 and to implementing an adult basic skills strategy by 2004.

The policies that are contributing to the achievement of these targets include:

- Standards Fund school improvement grant;
- Key Stage 3 strategy (providing extra support to pupils who start secondary school with achievement levels below their peers);
- Excellence in Cities programme (involving 58 LEAs from 2001) and Excellence Clusters (covering small areas of deprivation in a further 11 LEAs and including low-performing and more successful schools);
- Foundation Stage (a part of the National Curriculum focusing on child development from age three to end of primary school reception year);
- Early Excellence Centres (35 centres combining early learning and childcare);
- Education Action Zones (targeting disaffected pupils and aiming to raise standards);
- Extended Schools;
- Healthy Schools Programme (and National Healthy School Standard);

Table 4.6: DfES Objectives 1 and 2

	Delivery	Targets
Objective 1: Give children an excellent start in education so that they have a better foundation for future learning	**Under 5s:** Early years education (nursery places available to all three- and four-year-olds), national childcare strategy, neighbourhood nurseries, Sure Start	**Under 5s:** • Provide access to a free nursery place for every three-year-old whose parents want one, by 2004 • Provide childcare places for 1.6 million children by 2004 • Establish 100 Early Excellence Centres by 2004 • Establish 900 neighbourhood nurseries in disadvantaged areas by 2004 • Ensure that 500 Sure Start programmes will reach up to one third of young children in poverty and their families by 2004
	Primary school children: Literacy and numeracy strategies, enriched national curriculum, Children's Fund investment	**Primary school children:** • Increase percentage of 11-year-olds who achieve level 4 in each of Key Stage 2 English and maths tests beyond the targets for 2002, by 2004 • Narrow attainment gap by ensuring that there are no LEAs in which less than 65% of pupils achieve these standards (in English)
Objective 2: Enable all young people to develop and to equip themselves with the skills, knowledge and personal qualities needed for life and work	**Young people in secondary schools:** • National Key Stage 3 strategy (in literacy and numeracy) • Expansion of the Excellence in Cities programme (focusing on schools in the most deprived areas) • Expansion of Learning Support Units • Reformed school curriculum incorporating citizenship	**Young people in secondary schools:** • Ensure that 85% of 14-year-olds achieve level 5 of Key Stage 3 in English, maths, ICT and 80% in science, by 2007 • As milestones towards this target, 75% to achieve level 5 in English, maths and ICT and 70% in science, by 2004 • For 2004, as a minimum target, at least 65% to achieve level 5 in English and maths, and 60% in science in each LEA • Reduce from 25% to 15% by 2004, the proportion of pupils who do achieve at least one level 5 Key Stage 3 in English, maths or science • Ensure that all pupils who are excluded obtain an appropriate full-time education
	Meeting individual talents at 14 to 19: • Wider range of opportunities from age 14 by increasing vocational opportunities • Financial incentives and support to encourage young people to stay committed to learning • Support for young people in personal development through the Connexions service	**Meeting individual talents at 14 to 19:** • By 2004, increase by three percentage points the number of 19-year-olds achieving a qualification equivalent to NVQ level 2 compared to 2002 • Increase the proportion of 19-year-olds achieving a level 3 qualification from 51% in 2000 to 55% in 2004 • Implement the Connexions service nationally in 2002-03 • Ensure that there is an apprenticeship place for all who want one • Ensure every child leaving care is guaranteed access to education, training or a job

Source: DfES (2001)

- National Service Framework for Children (announced in February 2001);
- National Childcare Strategy;
- Quality Protects programme (for effective protection, better quality care and improved life chances for children looked after by local authorities);
- Sure Start (see below);
- Children's Fund (£380 million over three years to support interventions to prevent disaffection and social exclusion);
- Connexions (bridging education and work).

Progress

In terms of policies for the under-fives, the National Childcare Strategy has created over 380,000 new nursery places since 1997 (DWP, 2001, p 31). Funding for childcare has been mainly directed at 20% of the most disadvantaged areas through the Neighbourhood Nurseries initiative. This funding amounts to £203 million to 2004. Services for the under-fives also fall under Sure Start programmes.

In terms of primary school children, improvements in educational attainment for all ages have been achieved, especially in literacy and numeracy (Table 4.7).

Local measures of school performance may have encouraged schools to focus on children with average or above average ability, therefore changes to the average may not address inequalities. Floor targets are an important development (which are also evident in the national strategy for neighbourhood renewal (SEU, 2001) and *Opportunity for all* (DWP, 2002a) but, although welcome, these minima do not explicitly address inequalities. However, the DWP recognises that educational "standards will need to rise most quickly in disadvantaged areas if we are to narrow the gaps in attainment" (2001, p 46).

Table 4.7: Percentage of 11-year-olds achieving the expected standards (%)

	In 1997	In 2001	Target
Literacy	63	75	80
Numeracy	62	71	75

Source: DWP (2001, p 24)

Table 4.8: Evolution of Sure Start

Timetable	Programmes (number)	Coverage (number of children)
By 2000	59	49,000
By July 2001	191	140,000
By 2004	500	400,000

Sure Start initiative

Sure Start was established in June 1998 with a remit "to promote the physical, intellectual, social and emotional development of young children" and their families (DWP, 2001, p 42). It is a joint DoH/DfES unit with its own cross-cutting PSA, which was extended to cover 'childcare and early years' in the *2002 Spending Review* (see Appendix D). By 2004, it is expected that "about 80% [of children in Sure Start areas will] live in households with incomes less than half the national average". At its height, Sure Start will thus reach "about one third of all children aged under four living in poverty" (Sure Start, nd(a)).

Sure Start programmes have initially focused on geographical concentrations of children living in poverty. The ideal size of each programme is about 700 children, balancing economies of scale with a smaller number of children living in poverty. Geographical concentrations of more than 700 children (under four) who live in poverty are uncommon. Thus, "if Sure Start were to reach greater numbers of poor children, it would require progressively more programmes" (Sure Start, 2000, p 3).

Programmes focus on mainstream services (rather than introducing new ones), which may have wider applications in tackling health inequalities. As the further expansion of Sure Start programmes to cover more children in poverty is limited, the priority must be to improve mainstream services everywhere, especially for those children and families who live on the edge of poverty. Furthermore, as Sure Start services are available to all who live in the designated areas (not just children living in poverty), assessment of the uptake of services and of outcomes in Sure Start areas is essential to show if the approach is differentially benefiting the less well off in these areas of high concentrations of poverty and if the inequality gap is being reduced.

A report undertaken for the *2000 Spending Review* (Sure Start, 2000) found that:

- Sure Start spent about 2.4% of the £11.5 billion funding devoted to all services for the under-fives. The Sure Start budget will rise from £284 million in 2001-02 to £499 million in 2003-04.
- Progress had been made to improve services for under-fives which were "patchy, uncoordinated and of mixed quality".
- Programmes have engaged closely with parents and communities.
- Joint working between agencies was good.
- Demand for childcare in disadvantaged areas was not met.
- Few programmes had the capacity to deliver "sufficient pre-birth support".
- Sure Start should link better with services for children aged over four.

- The objective "to strengthen families and communities should place more emphasis on education and employment opportunities for parents".

The *2002 Spending Review* signalled an expansion of Sure Start by:

- "providing resources to create at least 250,000 childcare places";
- creating and operating children's centres in disadvantaged areas by combining the "responsibility for childcare, early years and Sure Start together in a single inter-departmental unit";
- "intending to simplify funding arrangements, streamline targets";
- guaranteeing a free early years education place for all three-year-olds whose parents want one (DfES PSA, 2002, see Appendix D, page 65).

Table 4.9: Sure Start objectives, PSAs and SDAs

Objective	PSA	SDA
Improving social and emotional development	• Reduce percentage of children aged 0-3 in 500 Sure Start areas who are re-registered within 12 months on child protection register by 20% by 2004	• All Sure Start areas to have agreed and implemented ways of caring and supporting mothers with postnatal depression • 100% of families with young children to have been contacted by local programmes within two months of birth
Improving health	• By 2004 in 500 Sure Start areas, 10% reduction in mothers who smoke in pregnancy	• Parenting support and information available to all parents • Local programmes to give guidance on breast-feeding and so on • 10% reduction in children in Sure Start areas children aged 0-3 admitted to hospital as emergency with gastro-enteritis, respiratory infection or severe injury
Improving children's ability to learn	• By 2004, 5% reduction in number of children with speech and language problems requiring specialist intervention by age 4.	• Increase use of libraries by parents with young children in Sure Start areas • All children to have access to good quality play and learning opportunities
Strengthening families and communities	• Reduce by 12% number of children aged 0-3 in Sure Start areas living in households in which no one is working	• 75% families reporting personal evidence of improvement in quality of services • All Sure Start to have parent representation • All Sure Start to have local targets for ensuring links between Sure Start and Jobcentres • All Sure Start to work with Early Years Development Care Plan to help close gap between availability of accessible childcare for children aged 0-3

Source: Sure Start (2001a)

Table 4.10: Local performance management of Sure Start programmes

	Period of assessment
Number of children under four living in Sure Start area that are reached by the programme, by population sub-group	Monthly
Progress towards PSA and SDA targets, measured against milestones	Quarterly
Progress towards PSA and SDA targets, measured against milestones	Annual
Updates of basic data	Annual
Updates on childcare places	Annual

Source: Sure Start (2001b)

The combined budget for childcare, early years education and Sure Start will be £1.5 billion.

Performance management of Sure Start recognises that benefits are expected to be evident in the long term and not necessarily in the PSA/SDA time-scale. SDA targets were considered as "reasonable measures of progress" of what programmes could be achieved between 2001-02 and 2003-04 (Sure Start, nd(b)) (see Table 4.9).

The combination of these shorter- and longer-term indicators of progress provides the framework for structure, process and outcome indicators that could be applied to other strategies tackling health inequalities.

Local performance management is included in the design of each programme from the outset (Table 4.10).

Conclusions

Most departmental targets support the government's overarching objectives to tackle health inequalities. Departmental systems and processes are shaped by the need to meet these objectives and targets. The new PSAs introduced in 2002 offer an increasingly coordinated approach to tackling health inequalities across government. Monitoring the achievement of targets and PSAs across departments could be improved, however, through two main mechanisms. First, a reporting mechanism such as the publication of an annual report could provide a regular and independent evaluation of progress. This report could be published under the auspices of a Select Committee or the Audit Commission. Second, health inequalities impact

assessments should be applied extensively within departments, as recommended by the Independent Inquiry and reinforced by the *2002 Cross-cutting Review* of health inequalities. Evidence of such assessments is currently sparse. In addition, efforts should be made to assess the likely impact on health inequalities at the time policy development is being considered. This is particularly important since it will not be possible to assess the impact of some policies for a number of years. When a policy change is being considered, information should be sought about any relevant existing (health) inequality – for example, poor access or educational attainment by particular social or ethnic groups – and efforts built into the policy to take account of this. The *Cross-cutting Review* recognised the need to make "information available where it is needed to support action, across the range of health inequalities dimensions including ethnic group, gender, age, disability etc" (HM Treasury/DoH, 2002, p 14) but how far this is possible with existing data is uncertain, particularly in relation to ethnic minorities. It is recommended that there should be a review of the relevant data collections and action taken to address any important limitations in these, either by changes to routine data collections or by commissioning studies, perhaps on a periodical basis, to provide the necessary information.

The key conclusions for performance management relating to policies tackling health inequality are:

- The government has stated the importance of tackling health inequalities by setting national targets. Without recognition in performance management systems and processes, health inequalities will get low priority.
- National targets have had more symbolic importance than practical significance so far but the results of the *2002 Spending Review*, *Cross-cutting Review* and forthcoming DoH delivery plan should establish targets tackling health inequalities on a more permanent basis.
- The two health inequality targets alone are insufficient. As the government recognises, they need to be supported by other indicators which:
  › incorporate the wider determinants of health;
  › support a joined-up approach;
  › are not simply disease-oriented;
  › are not dominated by healthcare/the NHS; and
  › leave scope for local and national priorities.

- Departments are supplementing average performance measures with minimum standards and degrees of variation. Even though audit processes such as health inequalities impact assessments are relatively rare, the inclusion of minima and variations within performance management is welcome, as is the *Cross-cutting Review* conclusion that "where appropriate, challenging floor targets should be set to level up service quality and outcomes" (HM Treasury/DoH, 2002, p 12).
- Standard definitions across departments aid coordination but the collation of data remains reliant on departmental systems.
- national levels.
- The *2002 Cross-cutting Review* proposal that DA(SER) should oversee the long-term strategy is an important step in the recognition of a need for a clear, cross-government ownership of policies at the national level.

This position needs to be developed further with regard to the infrastructure supporting the *Cross-cutting Review*'s proposals. It is recommended that:

The DA(SER) should:

- be supported either by a unit consisting of officials drawn from relevant departments or a clearly identified group of officials from those departments who work together to exchange information and produce material for it;
- address tax and benefit policy within its remit;
- be a long-standing, not a short-term committee and develop a rolling programme of work to tackle health inequalities.

The supporting unit should:

- track progress on tackling health inequalities as identified during the monitoring of the relevant departmental PSAs and targets and the basket of indicators;
- advise on further action (such as the addition of new targets and objectives);
- act as a source of information and advice to departments on the data available to analyse the impact of health inequalities on policy proposals and for health inequalities impact assessments.

The DA(SER) should produce an annual report for Parliament on progress in tackling health inequalities. Given the need to establish and maintain a cross-governmental ownership for the policy it is recommended that, perhaps on an experimental basis initially, a special cross-departmental Select Committee is formed, drawn from relevant Departmental Select Committees in order to receive an annual report and to question ministers on it.

5

Policy case study: the role of transport in tackling health inequalities

Links between transport and health inequalities

Transport has long been recognised as a contributory factor in exacerbating health inequalities. Such effects are manifest through pollution, injuries and poor access to employment, education, social networks and healthcare. The contribution of transport to alleviating health inequalities illustrates the need to address problems across government departments and across the life span.

The Independent Inquiry

The Acheson Report concluded that:

Lack of transport may damage health by denying access to people, goods and services. Furthermore, transport may damage health directly, most notably through accidental injury and air pollution. (Acheson, 1998, p 55)

The Report identified five way of tackling health inequalities through transport strategies.

Improving public transport

Recommendation 14: "We recommend the further development of a high quality public transport which is integrated with other forms of transport and is affordable to the user".

Encouraging walking and cycling

Recommendation 15: "We recommend further measures to encourage walking and cycling as forms of transport and to ensure the safe separation of pedestrians and cyclists from motor vehicles".

Reducing the use of motor vehicles

Recommendation 16: "We recommend further steps to reduce the usage of motor vehicles to cut mortality and morbidity associated with motor vehicle emissions".

Reducing traffic speed

Recommendation 17: "We recommend further measures to reduce traffic speed, by environmental design and modification of roads, lower speed limits in built up areas, and stricter enforcement of speed limits".

Making public transport affordable for pensioners and disadvantaged groups

Recommendation 18: "We recommend concessionary fares should be available to pensioners and disadvantaged groups throughout the country, and that local schemes should emulate high quality schemes, such as those in London and the West Midlands".

Transport, health inequalities and policies

Social and economic life has been shaped by transport. For example, about three quarters of all households now own at least one car; it is the most popular mode of transport across all income groups. For example, travel accounts for 17% (roughly £62) of weekly household expenditure with the majority of this (£52) being spent on motoring (DfT, 2001, p 93).

The lack of transport and/or lack of access to services disproportionately affects the lower socioeconomic groups, women, ethnic minority groups, children, older people and the mobility impaired. Less than 45% of unskilled manual and economically inactive households have a car; only 18% households (aged over 65, living alone) own a car (DTLR, 2000).

Transport policies can be classified as either 'health promoting' or 'health damaging' (HDA, 1998) (Table 5.1).

Transport policies to tackle health inequalities

The Integrated Transport White Paper (DETR, 1998) has set the context for recent policy development. It concluded that "the way we travel is making us a less healthy nation" and set the framework for:

- reducing pollution from transport;
- improving air quality;
- encouraging healthier lifestyles;
- reducing noise from transport;
- improving transport safety for users.

Specific policies have followed the White Paper and these are listed in Table 5.2.

Some of the national developments are explored below in more detail.

PSAs and targets

The DfT's PSAs (2002, see Appendix D, page 66) include targets that have impacts on transport and health inequalities (see Appendix D).

Sustainable development policies form part of DEFRA's PSA. These policies cover many wider determinants of health including transport, housing, planning, health and safety, and local government strategies. It aims to:

- advance social progress which recognises the needs of everyone;
- maintain high and stable levels of economic growth and employment.

The transport-related indicators cover dimensions such as education (how children get to school), geography (access to services in rural areas) and physical exercise (participation in sport and cultural activities) (see Appendix D).

Air pollution

The national air quality strategy (2000) set targets to reduce the risks of eight main air pollutants and particles to health. The government proposed its responsibilities for air quality as:

- providing a clear and simple policy framework;
- setting realistic and challenging objectives;
- creating regulatory and financial incentives;
- analysing costs and benefits;
- conducting monitoring and research.

Table 5.1: The effects of transport on health

Health promoting	Health damaging
• Enabling access to employment, shops, recreation, social support networks, health services, countryside • Recreation • Physical activity	• Pollution: particulate matter, nitrogen oxides, carbon monoxide, hydrocarbons, ozone, lead, benzene • Traffic injuries • Noise and vibration • Stress and anxiety • Danger • Loss of land and planning blight • Severance of communities by roads

Table 5.2: Selected transport policies that might affect health inequalities

Policy	Aim/target
A New Deal for Transport: Better for everyone (DETR, 1998)	White Paper contains section entitled 'Better health', which set the policy framework and targets.
'Rural bus challenge'	To stimulate new ideas in provision and promote rural public transport. £239 million (2001-02 to 2003-04). A similar scheme has been introduced for urban areas.
Local Transport Plans	Local authorities (in England, outside London) devise five-year plans that reflect local needs. They should be consistent with national policy objectives including promoting integrated transport, accessibility and safety. Investment will be delivered through LSPs and neighbourhood renewal strategies. "Improved accessibility planning and coordination between public transport providers will take account of health inequalities..." (HM Treasury, 2002, p 74).
National air quality strategy (1999)	To reduce exacerbation of asthma and reduce risks to those with chronic breathing and heart conditions.
1995 Disability Discrimination Act	To ensure all future public transport is accessible to older and disabled people.
Strategy for sustainable development (1999)	To advance social progress which recognises the needs of everyone.
Transport 2010 (2000)	DETR's 10-year plan for transport (July 2000)
2000 Transport Act	Introduced Regulatory Impact Assessment.
	Gave powers to local authorities to introduce Home Zones and Quiet Lanes.
	Equalisation of retirement age (making 1million men (aged 60-64) eligible for local authority concessionary fares).
School Travel Advisory Group (2000)	To support safe and healthy travel to school; to make better use of resources devoted to statutory school transport.
Tomorrow's roads: Safer for everyone (DTLR, 2000)	'Challenging targets reductions' in the number of people killed or seriously injured, to be reached by 2010.
Transport Direct (2001)	Scheme to allow people to plan their journeys, covering all types of travel. Involves planning, booking and real-time performance. To be implemented by 2003.
Cross-cutting Review on health inequalities (2001-02) (HM Treasury/ DoH, 2002)	To analyse the impact of transport (among other things) on health.
Free bus pass	Guaranteed free bus pass for older and disabled people in England and Wales since June 2001.
Making the connections: Transport and social exclusion (SEU, 2002)	The Social Exclusion Unit's interim report published in May 2002.
Fuel Duty Rebate (May 2002)	Extension of rebate for transport services provided by non-profit making community transport bodies.
DfT PSA target	"Reduce the number of peoples killed or seriously injured in GB in road accidents by 40% and the number of children killed or seriously injured by 50%, by 2010 compared with the average for 1994-98, tackling the significantly higher incidence in disadvantaged communities" (HM Treasury, 2002, p 72).

The NAO (2001b) endorsed this approach but advised that DEFRA should:

- take stock of gaps in knowledge of health effects of air pollution;
- recognise and respond to the scope for future air quality to differ from forecast levels;
- improve consultation processes.

The NAO recommended that:

- membership of expert panels should be widened;
- a timetable for reviews of air quality standards should be established;
- cost-benefit analysis to inform assessment of air quality policy proposals should be considered;
- local authorities' progress should be reviewed.

DoH consultation results on the delivery plan

The results of the consultation exercise were published in June 2002 (DoH, 2002b). Transport was considered as a wider determinant of health: "lack of transport is one barrier to poor people gaining access to core services and leisure activities" (DoH, 2002b, p 21). Suggested improvements included:

- encouraging LSPs to focus on transport;
- ensuring access to open space;
- reducing the higher risk to child pedestrians in poorer neighbourhoods;
- developing links between community safety and health.

The consultation results included reference to road safety in terms of the "higher risk to child pedestrians" (DoH, 2002b, p 21) but air quality was not mentioned. (By contrast, air quality was mentioned in *From vision to reality* (DoH, 2001a) but transport was largely absent.)

SEU report on transport and social exclusion

The report (SEU, 2002) argued that transport can be a result of social exclusion or reinforce it. It identified the main barriers to work, learning and healthcare as access, availability, cost and limited travel horizons. The report offered strategies to overcome barriers including objectives and target setting, planning integration, funding and

performance management, improving access and availability, addressing cost barriers, widening travel horizons and reducing the need to travel. However, several barriers to success are also evident; the report claims that social costs have hitherto not be given due weight in transport policy, that there is fragmented and inequitable funding, and that regulatory barriers remain.

Cross-cutting Review

The purpose of the HM Treasury's *Cross-cutting Review* on health inequalities was:

> To analyse the impact on *health* of poverty, employment, education, crime, *transport*, fuel poverty and related factors, and assess and improve the mechanisms for tackling these problems. (HM Treasury, 2001; emphasis added)

Moreover, the review's conclusions made little reference to transport per se but recommended an "expansion of initiatives to raise the level of physical activity in disadvantaged communities" (HM Treasury/DoH, 2002, p 158).

The report of the *Cross-cutting Review* did, however, recognise the link both to deprivation and to geographical inequalities in health resulting from inequalities in provision of, and access to, transport services (HM Treasury/DoH, 2002, p 50). It pointed to the importance of transport and the need for "improving accessibility of disadvantaged groups to core facilities (such as public services and retail outlets), through improved mainstream and targeted public transport links and through better land use planning" (p 13).

In the remainder of this chapter, two specific national policies are explored in further detail: access and mobility, and child road safety policy.

Access and mobility

Transport facilitates access for people rather than being an end in itself. Transport difficulties (such as the absence of services, their poor quality and cost) pose major barriers for people to access healthcare services, employment, food (for a healthy diet) and social networks. It is thus vital to the reduction of health inequalities.

Problem

Access via transport is closely related to inequalities across all social categories, and mirrored in ownership of and access to cars, and use of public transport. Social class, geography and age are illustrated here.

Social class

Nearly one third of households do not own a car (SEU, 2002) but this varies significantly by social class – a pattern which has changed slightly in recent years (Figure 5.1).

There is a heavy reliance on public transport for lower income groups, for example, 7% of people without cars have missed, turned down or chosen not to seek medical help in the last year because of transport problems (which is twice the rate of the overall population) (SEU, 2002).

Geography

The 1991 Census found that, in rural areas, only 15% had no access to a car (compared with 34% in urban areas). Nonetheless, only 23% used public transport in rural areas if they had no car (compared with 49% in urban areas), reflecting the low supply of rural transport. Deprived areas are particularly affected by transport difficulties, for example, in the poorest 10% of wards, half of households do not own a car. Also, one in ten people in low-income areas have turned down a job in the last year because of transport difficulties (SEU, 2002). It is therefore recommended that departments share such data on access to help improve the uptake of healthcare and employment opportunities.

Age

The most significant barriers to mobility for older people relate to physical difficulties. Their concerns also centre on information, access and cost (DETR, 2001a). For example, access is made difficult by poor infrastructure and only a fifth of buses meet accessibility requirements (SEU, 2002). Mobile individuals in households with a car travel up to 12 times further each year than a person with mobility problems in a household with no car (Table 5.3).

Households comprising older people have lower rates of car ownership: while 61% of householders aged between 65 and 74 own a car, this figure falls to 35% and 22% for those aged over 75 and those over 64 living alone, respectively (HDA, 1998).

Figure 5.1: Household car ownership by income quintile (1989–1991 and 1998–2000)

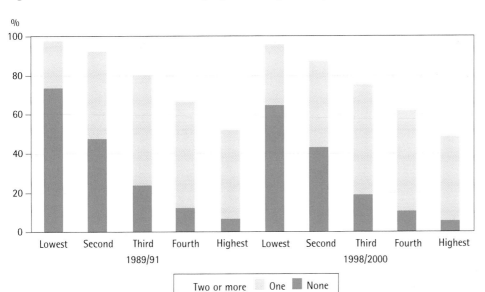

Source: DfT (2001, p 9)

Table 5.3: Average distance travelled (in miles) per person (by age group) per year (1996–98)

	Households with no car		Households with car(s)	
	No mobility problem	Some mobility difficulty	No mobility problem	Some mobility difficulty
0-16 years	1,550		4,442	
17-29	3,665	2,008	8,997	5,741
30-49	3,738	2,745	10,457	6,615
50-64	3,066	1,533	9,357	6,615
65-79	2,610	1,805	5,890	4,632
80+	2,049	880	4,079	2,103

Source: DETR (2000)

Overall, the UK faces a situation in which public transport fares are more expensive, bus usage has been declining and levels of car use are high (despite lower car ownership) compared with other countries (SEU, 2002).

Policy

Transport policy and planning across government is integrating health inequality issues through:

- explicit policy development, as illustrated by the SEU study of transport and social exclusion;
- funding of specific programmes such as community transport advisory service (for example, dial-a-ride schemes);
- more implicit means such as sponsoring research into the transport needs of different groups. Such initiatives help generate guidance for service operators.

In each mechanism, the levers of change are finance, guidance and legislation. However, transport funding is marked by inequity and fragmentation (SEU, 2002). For example, the 10-year transport plan is skewed towards transport used by high income individuals; it aims to allocate 11% of its £120 billion to buses compared with 40% for passenger rail (SEU, 2002). Responsibility is fragmented between different departments. For example, revenue support for buses is directed through three separate streams within DfT. Also, "in addition to the £1 billion DTLR spends on buses, a further £900 million is spent on school, patients and social services transport" (SEU, 2002, para 4.12). No single department is responsible for improving access to work, learning or healthcare.

Older people

A focus on older people illustrates many of the difficulties in improving access and mobility. Older people report high levels of difficulty in gaining access to all modes of transport. A DETR report (2001a) made a 'general' recommendation for a "national uniform scheme for concessionary fares".

The Independent Inquiry noted that over 10 million people are eligible for concessionary fares. As schemes and services vary, the uptake of these schemes is lower in areas of low population density (Acheson, 1998, p 90). In line with the Inquiry's recommendation (No 18), concessionary fares have been made available to older people. Concessionary fares apply to all older people (rather than being targeted at those on low incomes) and are estimated to cost the government £470 million per annum (SEU, 2002). Prompted largely by the equalisation of the entitlement age for reduced fares (under the 2000 Transport Act, up to 1 million men (aged 60-64) will benefit. The cost to bus operators (who are reimbursed by the local authority for the revenue foregone) is cost-neutral but its overall cost is expected to cost £50 million per annum (DTLR, 2001a).

A recent survey revealed that:

- 59% of people over 60 own a concessionary fare pass (compared with 11% who own a Senior Railcard);
- concessionary fare pass ownership is widespread among women, people from minority ethnic groups, non-drivers and those from C2, D and E households;

- people with any type of impairment are slightly less likely to have a bus pass than those without impairment;
- 75% pay 25 pence or less per trip with 40% travelling free;
- possession of a bus pass results in 37% of holders making more trips (DTLR, 2001b).

The 2000 Transport Act enables local authorities to introduce concessionary schemes and to vary the amount of concession. Concessions can also be offered to other groups of people (such as children) or on other modes of transport (such as taxis). A DTLR (2002) survey monitored the impact of the Transport Act and found that:

- 94% of local authorities offer a half-fare concessionary scheme for older people, 90% for disabled people and 60% for people who are registered blind;
- two million people live in areas offering free travel;
- 27% of local authorities had a concessionary fare scheme for school children.

Progress

Policies relating to mobility (and especially older people) have been implemented, which seek to improve the affordability, availability and accessibility of transport. These are in line with the Inquiry's recommendations. Despite an acceptable definition of basic minimum access (DETR, 2000), the importance of impact assessments is recognised in transport.

A higher uptake of concessionary fares will enable older people (especially those who are mobility-impaired or socially isolated) to access services. Greater awareness of entitlements through information availability and publicity campaigns would aid their uptake but must be accompanied by improvements to service provision (for example, coordination of services) and travel information (DTLR, 2001b) – the national Transport Direct telephone service should aid this. The SEU (2002) recommends that concessionary fares should also be introduced for other groups including jobseekers, lone parents and people receiving the Employment Tax Credit; the 2000 Transport Act allows for this. Also, the report highlights the anomaly that community transport providers are ineligible to receive concessionary fare income;

their passengers have to pay whereas those on mainstream transport travel free or half-price.

Further, substantial barriers remain in coordinating initiatives to improve access, as identified by a JRF (2001) report:

- high costs of fares;
- inadequacy of routes;
- poor vehicular access;
- poor training and inadequate staffing;
- personal safety and security.

Children and road safety

Problem

Road safety issues impinge on health inequalities, especially for children. There is a direct relationship with injury and deaths, and an indirect relationship in terms of perceived dangers and restricted social interaction.

Direct impacts are evident in casualties and deaths:

- In 2001, 3,450 people were killed in road traffic accidents, 1% more than in 2000 (DfT, 2002).
- Direct costs of injuries and deaths are about £3 billion annually (DTLR, 2000).
- "28 more children were killed on the roads in 2001 than in 2000, an increase of 15" (DfT, 2002).
- "Pedestrian casualties fell by 3% between 2000 and 2001 and the number of people killed or seriously injured pedestrians was down by 5%" (DfT, 2002).
- Children from minority ethnic groups are at a "substantially increased risk of pedestrian injury" in the UK; "children of Asian ethnic origin appear to be disproportionately vulnerable" (DETR, 2001b, p 1).
- The child (0-14 years) pedestrian fatality rate (per 100,000) in Great Britain was 0.9 in 2000 compared with 0.7 in France and 0.5 in Germany (DfT, 2002).

The Independent Inquiry identified the health inequalities relating to children in terms of traffic and pedestrian accidents. However, it made no specific recommendation about children's safety, rather it sought "further measures to encourage walking and cycling" and the "safe separation of pedestrian and cyclists from motor vehicles" (Recommendation 15). The Inquiry noted that "pedestrian injury death rates for children in social class V are five times higher than those in social class I, and are higher for boys than girls" (Acheson, 1998, p 57). This inequality was later cited by the government in its 'Quality of Life' indicators (1999). The Inquiry estimated 600 fewer deaths among men (aged 20-64) each year if all groups experienced death rates from motor vehicles traffic accidents currently experienced in social classes I and II combined (p 60).

Indirect impacts (such as perceived dangers and reduced interaction) are also evident. These are felt across all groups and ages (in terms of reduced activity levels, for example). Children are especially affected in terms of lower levels of independent travel and activity.

Policy

Tomorrow's roads (DTLR, 2000) outlined the policy interventions (addressing children), which have sought to influence traffic speed, safer travel on bicycles and travel to school. These included:

* targets for reductions in death and injury;
* traffic calming and speed reductions;
* road safety education and campaigns;
* school travel programmes.

At the time the report was published these initiatives were being implemented. The implementation of two further policies was scheduled for the "next 2-3 years":

* monitoring high risk groups and exploring ways of improving their safety;
* developing programmes which promote child pedestrian training schemes in deprived areas.

Targets

The introduction of measures has helped to meet the previous target (road casualty reduction of one third by 2000, set in 1987) for all groups. While reductions of 39% in road deaths and of 45% in serious injuries have been achieved, the rate for accidents and slight injuries has not declined greatly (DTLR, 2000).

The *Tomorrow's roads* document set targets for 2010:

* 40% reduction in the number of people killed or seriously injured in road accidents;
* 50% reduction in the number of children killed or seriously injured in road accidents;
* 10% reduction in the 'slight casualty rate' (number of people slightly injured per 100 million vehicle kilometres).

These targets have been refined by the *2002 Spending Review*. One of DfT's PSA targets is to:

Reduce the number of people killed or seriously injured in GB in road accidents by 40% and the number of children killed or seriously injured by 50%, by 2010 compared with the average for 1994-98, tackling the significantly higher incidence in disadvantaged communities. (HM Treasury, 2002, p 72)

Progress is apparent in 2001 figures although the target relating to children is still challenging:

the number of people killed or seriously injured was 15% below the 1994-98 average; the number of children killed or seriously inured was 27% below the 1994-98 average; and the slight casualty rate was 6% below the 1994-98 average. (DfT, 2002)

These targets are closely connected with English and Scottish public health strategies but need to be monitored regularly through formal mechanisms such as the routine monitoring of PSAs and targets.

Calming and speed reduction

Children are expected to benefit from various road safety measures proposed in *Tomorrow's roads*. Some measures such as traffic calming will disproportionately benefit children. Local authorities have powers under the 2000 Transport Act to introduce 20mph zones, especially around schools and residential areas. Evidence shows a 5% drop in accidents for every 1mph reduction in speed (Crombie, 2002).

Road safety education

Road safety education is promoted for different groups:

- *Babies and very young children:* advising parents and teachers on protection in cars and teaching safe behaviour on the road.
- *Primary age children:* providing child pedestrian and cycle training schemes and alerting parents to risk.
- *Older children:* providing road safety information as children go on longer journeys.
- *Older teenagers:* providing advice as they contemplate more independent mobility.

As most casualties occur when children travel further and more independently (for example, to secondary schools), the emphasis of interventions should be on such groups (Laflamme and Engstrom, 2002).

Road safety for children has been introduced into the personal, social and health education curriculum at Key Stages 1 and 2 (ages 5-11). The DTLR and DfES have undertaken joint work to assist schools to incorporate road safety effectively into the curriculum. The government thus aims to "continue to encourage schools to teach road safety" (DTLR, 2000, p 20). However, this aspect of the curriculum is not yet compulsory.

School travel programmes

Travel to school poses particular difficulties. Nearly 20% of cars on the road in urban areas at the morning peak (8.50am) are taking children to school. About a fifth of pedestrian casualties occur en route to school. Such figures are exacerbated by the rise in school journeys taken by car, which has risen from 16% to 30% in the last 10 years. The length of such journeys has also risen (DTLR/DfES/DOH, 2002).

In response, several policy initiatives have been introduced. For example, the School Travel Advisory Group (STAG) was established in December 1998 and reported to Ministers in January 2000; it recommended:

- minimum standard for concessionary child bus fares;

- more road safety education;
- better enforcement of speed restrictions.

STAG drew its membership from the DETR, DfEE and DoH. The group disseminated best practice and sought to highlight school travel issues within local authorities.

Progress

Progress is evident in process and outcome measures. A national coordinator has been appointed for child pedestrian training in deprived areas. The Highways Agency has developed and implemented 'child-friendly areas' on trunk roads near schools and in residential areas. The impact has, however, been 'inconclusive' due to the low number of accidents involving children in these areas. Road safety audits have been included in guidance for new local transport plans (DETR, 2001b). Also, £3.5 million was awarded to 28 local authorities for child safety road projects in 2001.

Progress has been made in reducing child deaths and injuries. In 2000, 39,715 children were killed or injured on roads, of which 22,400 were pedestrians or cyclists (DfT, 2002), representing a 14% reduction in the number of children killed on UK roads (since 1999). However, the number of child pedestrian deaths showed no change (107 deaths) over this period. Improvements among 10- to 15-year-olds have been less dramatic as reductions in the number of deaths and injuries have been smaller in this age group than others. Deaths and injuries to children aged under 16 years fell by 5% between 1999 and 2000 but for 10- to 15-year-olds, this fall was only 2% (DTLR, 2000). Process and outcome indicators (such as these) need to form part of the widespread health inequalities impact assessment because, for example, children from ethnic minorities have higher casualty rates (DETR, 2001b).

School transport schemes could be developed to support these initiatives. Entitlement to free school transport misses some children from low-income families who may need assistance. Spare capacity on school buses is often unused and may not meet accessibility standards (making them redundant for other groups at other times). The SEU (2002) advocates further developments with regard to children and road safety, particularly in reducing inequalities in child pedestrian accidents between deprived communities and the national average.

Conclusions

Transport policies may reduce or exacerbate health inequalities. The examples of access and mobility, and child safety strategies illustrate the possible positive and negative impacts on health inequalities.

The SEU (2002) also made recommendations for tackling social exclusion with regard to transport:

- clearer accountability for improving outcomes through accessibility and impact planning;
- greater flexibility to achieve outcomes;
- joined-up and better targeted resources;
- improved skills, expertise and capacity to consult communities and assess their needs;
- better targeting for specific activities (such as work, learning and healthcare);
- reductions in the need to travel (mainly through land-use planning).

The London Health Commission (2001) assessed the health impact of the Mayor's draft transport strategy and recommended that it should:

- promote modes of transport other than motor vehicles;
- link transport, economic development and spatial development;
- redress social inequalities;
- avoid community severance;
- link proposals for the greatest benefit to health;
- segregate modes of transport;
- involve local authorities;
- develop baseline statistics and targets for health gain.

Using these recommendations, some conclusions can be drawn.

Promote modes of transport other than motor vehicles

Public transport is largely inadequate for the basic needs of most people (except in some central areas of large cities) (JRF, 2001; SEU,

2002). Improvements to availability, affordability and accessibility are required, but such barriers may be insurmountable in rural areas where car ownership is often deemed necessary given the shortcomings of public transport. The promotion of buses through better targeting of existing resources can improve access for vulnerable groups. A review of support mechanisms for buses was heralded as part of the *2002 Spending Review* (HM Treasury, 2002). Transport should be an important consideration in the remit of the DA(SER) in its oversight of the strategy on health inequalities.

Social inequalities and community severance

Policies to encourage economic regeneration can widen social inequalities (through pollution and congestion) which are felt especially in poor neighbourhoods. Policies to promote sustainable development and reduce inequality are therefore positive. Transport needs to be integrated into such strategies but compromises between transport, sustainable development and inequalities appear likely:

Policies which aim to mitigate the environmental impacts of traffic may sometimes come into conflict with the social inclusion of low-income and other disadvantaged groups and communities. (JRF, 2001, p 1)

The consequences of these various policies need to be monitored more closely, for example through health inequalities impact assessments.

Involvement of local authorities

Local transport plans and local authorities' powers can help to reduce road casualties and improve child safety. Local authorities still face difficulties in contributing fully to this agenda including lack of clear responsibility for improving access, regulatory barriers that impede effective solutions, fragmented and inequitable funding, and a lack of institutional skills and capacity (SEU, 2002). Moreover, "many of the problems associated with poor transport and accessibility for low income and other disadvantaged groups are beyond the capacity of local authorities to resolve" (JRF, 2001). The JRF report cited the following reasons:

- limited resources;
- insufficient powers;
- problems of retaining and/or providing basic local transport services in low-income areas;
- conflicting intentions and competing priorities of central government policies within and between departments;
- insufficient guidance.

Mechanisms such as LSPs and HImPs should foster the involvement of other partners to deliver transport improvements, and it is recommended that health inequalities should be included within the remit of local authorities' scrutiny committees to aid local implementation.

Targets, monitoring and impact assessment

It is a positive development that various targets have been set in relation to transport but they must be accompanied by mechanisms to evaluate their impact in relation to child pedestrian accidents and pollution (SEU, 2002). The need for 'social equity audits' and health inequalities impact assessments thus remains high (SEU, 2002). These assessments should be applied across all areas, including concessionary fares and child casualties. Indeed, the government recommends that local authorities should assess the equity implications of their transport policies, adjusting policies where necessary. These assessments should also apply to central government policies.

6

Discussion and interpretation

Discussion of emergent themes

This study has tracked the development of policies on health inequalities since the publication of the Independent Inquiry and has identified five dimensions that characterise the progress made and the work that remains. They are:

- activity related to tackling health inequalities;
- policy-making developments across government;
- systems to support policies;
- embedding policies within structure and processes;
- measuring and monitoring progress.

This chapter considers each of these in order to set policy developments in context, explain the state of progress and suggest how policies might tackle health inequalities in future. Further possible interpretations are provided later in this chapter.

Significant amount of activity related to tackling health inequalities

The Independent Inquiry certainly helped to raise the profile of health inequalities across government and provided the basis for policy development. The impact of the report on policy:

- prompted new policies to tackle health inequalities;
- introduced a health inequality dimension to existing policies;
- encouraged or contributed to a climate of opinion in favour of tackling health inequalities;

- acted as a source book or reference against which policies can be examined and tested.

Some recommendations have not resulted in action thus far (for example, water fluoridation, reform of private practice and of the Common Agricultural Policy).

Policies to tackle health inequalities are evident across the life span and focus on children and families, in line with the key recommendations of the Acheson Report. They have, however, tended to focus on discrete geographical areas. These area-based policies focus on concentrations of poverty but may miss 'poor' individuals living in more affluent areas and do not, therefore, deal with the problem effectively. The need to "reach more than the most deprived areas" was recognised in the *2002 Cross-cutting Review* (HM Treasury/DoH, 2002, p 2) and so its emphasis on the need for "national health inequalities targets to be embedded in and delivered through mainstream programmes across Government" (HM Treasury/DoH, 2002, p 12) was most welcome. Individually-based policies (such as tax credits), which form part of the government's welfare-to-work strategy and will tackle health inequalities universally, need to continue to be pursued as well, but need to be more 'joined up' with other relevant policies.

Policy-making developments across government

It is crucial that health inequalities have been recognised as not simply a matter for the DoH. Departments such as the DfES, DfT and DWP have made notable contributions to policy. The inclusion of health inequalities on the policy agenda across government has been underlined and strengthened by fiscal reforms and the HM

Treasury-led *Cross-cutting Review* of health inequalities. Through the Independent Inquiry and the government's public health strategy, departments have recognised their potential contribution to tackling health inequalities.

Up to 2001, a varied set of policies and initiatives were developed. Although they addressed most of the Inquiry's recommendations, there appeared relatively little coherence to them. They tended to be add-on or one-off initiatives, rather than influencing mainstream policy, planning or provision. Since 2001, a more systematic approach across government is evident via:

- two national health inequality targets;
- the DoH report *From vision to reality* (2001a);
- the HM Treasury's *Cross-cutting Review* of health inequalities (HM Treasury/DoH, 2002);
- the DoH *Consultation on a plan for delivery* (2001b).

These strengthen existing structures and processes and imply a maturation of policy across government. They reflect the increasing recognition of the need to sustain a programme over a long period of time, to ensure that action across government at both national and local levels is coherent (or joined up), and that action needs to be embedded in mainstream structures and processes. These messages are evident in the *2002 Cross-cutting Review*. It is hoped that the forthcoming DoH delivery plan will include detailed proposals for the structures and processes likely to ensure effective implementation and on how health inequalities will be incorporated into mainstream policies in line with the *Cross-cutting Review*.

These departmental contributions presage a more firmly established and coherent approach across government to tackling health inequalities. The HM Treasury's own role, in conjunction with the DWP, in determining tax and benefit levels, has remained, however, outside this nexus. It is therefore recommended that these policies should be recognised as much a part of strategies to tackle health inequalities as others covering education, transport, housing and so on, and that joined-up government should also be applied in this area. These levels are crucial to tackling the living standards and income inequality that the Acheson Report highlighted as one of three crucial recommendations. This was reinforced by

the *2002 Cross-cutting Review* which stated: "Poverty and material disadvantage in all its forms, has a significant effect on health inequalities. There is strong evidence showing differential health outcomes by social class" (HM Treasury/DoH, 2002, p 31).

Since 2001, progress has been substantial. It remains to be seen whether this will be sustainable and whether health inequalities (and the wider determinants) will continue to secure priority within departments. Health inequality policies on departmental agendas are more secure and the ownership of the problem by policy makers more integrated in some departments than in others. If progress on tackling health inequalities is to be sustained alongside more pressing, high profile priorities and a cross-departmental ownership fostered, it must be built into appropriate systems and processes.

Policies supported by systems and processes

To ensure effective implementation in the long term, policies need to be embedded in the fabric of policy-making structures and processes. Mechanisms that are appropriate for tackling health inequalities include cross-cutting units, joint management, taskforces and targets.

Cross-cutting units (such as the SEU or PIU) synthesise data and provide analysis of policy problems. However, there is a danger that these horizontal mechanisms are not coordinated with departmental (vertical) structures and processes (Richards, 2001; Richards and Smith, 2002). Joint management is apparent in cross-departmental units such as Sure Start, which is run by a joint DfES-DoH unit, with its own targets relevant to tackling health inequalities. It reports to Ministers in both departments. The DoH has also convened the Inequalities and Public Health Taskforce to oversee the implementation of part of *The NHS Plan*, to consider health inequalities targets and to advise on the DoH's consultation. It is recommended that the remit of the Inequalities and Public Health Taskforce should be revised to examine and to promote ways in which a health inequality dimension can be embedded in mainstream policy, planning and provision in central government and at the local level.

The extensive range of targets operates at all organisational levels. PSAs are perhaps the most significant development as they shape systems and processes within and between departments; many PSAs could contribute to significant reductions in health inequalities (see Appendix D). These targets reinforce the position of health inequalities within departments. It is significant, therefore, that tackling health inequalities forms one of the DoH's PSAs (2002, see Appendix D, page 65). Health inequalities are also reflected in the national PSA for local government, according to the *2002 Spending Review*. Appropriate targets should also be included at the local level and action should be taken to ensure that local authority scrutiny committees include health inequalities within their remit. As the *2002 Cross-cutting Review* concludes:

> To be effective, interventions to tackle health inequalities need to have leadership at the local level and be accountable to local communities. The intention is to put in place delivery mechanisms and structures to empower those at local level to design and carry out the interventions most effective and appropriate for their communities to deliver the strategy. (HM Treasury/DoH, 2002, p 9)

Embedding health inequality policy within structures and processes

Policies have emphasised special projects and funding 'challenges', often through short-term, geographically-based initiatives. This innovation and experimentation has been useful but there is a danger that these initiatives remain marginal to, or are a substitute for, mainstream policy, planning or provision. Policy developments thus need to be spread more widely.

The *2002 Spending Review* recognised the need to mainstream health inequalities within the work of the NHS and DoH, DfES, DfT, DCMS, the Home Office, the ODPM, DWP and DEFRA. This recognition is an important and necessary development. It identified specific actions which are largely focused on 'deprived areas' and 'disadvantaged communities', notably in terms of resource allocation for the NHS and schools, smoking cessation services, programmes for children's nutrition, physical activity and housing

conditions (for families with young children and older people). While these are important areas, if the *Review* had amounted simply to these initiatives and the few amendments to PSAs, much of the earlier impetus would be lost. The *2002 Cross-cutting Review*, meanwhile, provides a more comprehensive approach to health inequalities. It provides a strategic framework, an acceptance of the need for action across government and analysis of the interventions needed to tackle the wider determinants.

In a report for the Neighbourhood Renewal Unit and Regional Coordination Unit, Stewart et al (2002) offer useful insights into the difficulties of mainstreaming. Thus far, mainstreaming has tended to be "piecemeal and opportunistic", taking "second place to the preparation of delivery plans and the implementation of programmes" (p 30), and dependent on being driven by central government. The report recommended incentives to foster mainstreaming:

- evaluation of what works for the mainstream;
- development of continuity strategies for initiatives;
- shared responsibility for exchange and dissemination between initiatives;
- input to and from initiatives and mainstream planning;
- design of programmes which stress innovation;
- links between senior officials of initiatives and mainstream programmes;
- links between targets for initiatives and those of mainstream programmes;
- incorporation of lessons from initiatives into performance management.

The lessons and methods can be applied and integrated with broader health inequality policy at national and local levels.

If a health inequality dimension can be introduced into mainstreamed programmes, the benefits could be significant. Targets and performance management will be crucial. It is therefore encouraging that health inequalities will be embedded in the NHS performance management framework and that it is being considered in local government performance management. The forthcoming delivery plan should cover this in detail. The DA(SER), which it is recommended should be supported by a cross-departmental group of officials, is to oversee the implementation of this long-term strategy. These mechanisms presage a more robust system for future policy implementation, which would seemingly overcome many of the problems of joined-up working identified in the *Wiring it up* report (PIU, 2000). However, close attention of audit and budgetary systems, and support for officials working across departments will still be required.

Measuring and monitoring progress

The DA(SER) aims to improve the coordination and targeting of mainstream services and to implement the long-term strategy. It will need to:

- be long standing (as 'quick wins' cannot be expected);
- have a rolling programme of action;
- have good quality data on which to assess progress;
- understand the measurement difficulties relating to health inequalities.

Measuring progress policies in tackling health inequalities is problematic because:

- the relationship between policy and health outcomes is uncertain;
- changes in health inequality can rarely be attributed to specific policies;
- the most suitable combination of policies to tackle health inequalities is unknown;
- little is known about the unintended consequences of policies or the role of the wider socioeconomic context.

As the *2002 Cross-cutting Review* acknowledged, the evidence base for policies to tackle health inequalities is mixed, with more information available on single risk factors than the "more complex, multi-factorial socio-economic and environmental determinants" (p 23). Despite the ongoing work of the Health Development Agency (HDA), research on which interventions are effective in reducing health inequalities is needed. Central departments may wish to commission this, either collectively or in relation to their own responsibilities, but, in either case, the outcomes should be shared. Moreover, there is also a strong case for independent evaluation. Given the cross-sectoral nature of the problem, there is as much need for collaboration and data sharing within the research community as within central government. It is therefore recommended that the ESRC and MRC consider creating a centre of expertise to conduct and collate studies that describe and explain effective interventions to tackle health inequalities. This might also act as a forum for funding agencies involved in health inequalities research to coordinate research programmes which focus on outcomes (rather than causation which is relatively well established).

The national health inequality targets have provided an important symbolic function but are being revised to make them meaningful in the light of changes to the NHS structures and the recording of social class data. It is important that data underpinning the new targets (and performance management) are shared between and are relevant to agencies at the local and national levels. There should be a review of the data to ensure that it covers all relevant factors and groups that require monitoring in relation to health inequalities, notably social class, birth registrations by lone parents and in relation to ethnic minorities. The 'basket' of indicators (to be published in 2003) should play a practical role in helping to measure the results of policy interventions. It will be important to develop a manageable set of indicators that adequately measure performance over the wide range of policies and services involved. Given the long time-scales involved in tackling health inequalities, it is recommended that indicators include interim measures to track progress in establishing structures and processes as well as longer-term ones to appraise outcomes.

While interim (output) markers are beginning to emerge from programmes such as Sure Start, health outcomes are not yet apparent. Extant data cannot be attributed to specific policy changes, as yet. These data can, however, be shared and used more effectively, once their inadequacies have been overcome. The time lag between policy making, implementation and outcomes needs to be recognised and underlines the need for intermediate progress indicators as part of performance management indicators. These 'progress' indicators should include process indicators (such as time-scales for partnership formation) and interim targets (such as uptake rates of services for vulnerable groups).

Health inequalities impact assessments are the means of monitoring the results of policy interventions and generating the evidence to ensure that policies are not inadvertently widening health inequalities. Impact assessments have been widely introduced but these invariably neglect inequalities. Most policies have not been accompanied by health inequalities impact assessment: even though it was one of the three crucial recommendations in the Independent Inquiry and despite the work of the HDA, the use of such assessments is still patchy across departments. The national health inequality targets, targets in education and employment, and the proposed reduction of inequality regarding pollution and child pedestrian accidents (SEU, 2002) indicate progress, but further work remains. Departments should give greater emphasis to (health) inequality impact assessment by framing their targets with an inequality dimension and improving institutional capacity (such as data availability) and individual skills (such as staff training).

Interpreting progress

These dimensions provide a descriptive analysis of progress in tackling health inequalities but they lack an explanatory framework within which recent progress or developments in the future can be evaluated. A framework can also aid identification of the points of leverage within the policy-making machinery. As tackling health inequalities across government remains relatively new, a broader framework and explanation is valuable as it helps to gauge strengths and weaknesses of specific programmes and the general policy direction. It also provides lessons to others.

Bull and Hamer (2001) summarised the components of effective policy development with regard to health inequalities (Table 6.1). An alternative approach involves seven phases through which policy making might move (Table 6.2). The Independent Inquiry played a crucial role in shaping the agenda and providing direction for subsequent policies, and a wide range of initiatives related to tax and benefit reforms and to transport have been introduced. These, and other areas, are being supported by an increasingly robust performance management system. Progress is, however, less apparent in

mainstreaming the methods and lessons of short-term and area-based initiatives, in monitoring progress and in being able to identify the (health) outcomes. Both interpretations offer a linear, rationalistic interpretation that is limiting; they do not provide explanations of how or why change was or might be possible.

A third interpretation helps to explain how change is generated; it draws on a model of policy making – the *policy window* model (Kingdon, 1995; Exworthy et al, 2002). This model assumes that policy-making processes comprise three streams (problem, policy and politics) that must be joined for change to occur. Certain conditions are required for this:

- *problem stream:* evidence must be plausible;
- *policy stream:* interventions must be feasible;
- *politics stream:* values and vision must be compatible.

Once joined, the policy window is open. Unless they are joined or when they are separated, the window is closed and change is less likely.

The *problem stream* consists of issues that need to be defined as problems amenable to policy interventions. For a long time, health inequalities were not defined as a problem. The Independent Inquiry and other evidence have established health inequalities as a 'policy problem' which has now been accepted by government. Evidence of the problem must therefore be plausible to generate action. The *policy stream* comprises strategies and initiatives which must be technically feasible, congruent with the dominant (sociopolitical) values and anticipate future constraints (such as lower tax revenues). The policy stream must comprise appropriate systems and processes (such as performance management). While there are some concerns about the feasibility of some policies and their future constraints, policies generally do match with the government's values and objectives. However, there may be a tension between approaches that adopt a social gradient across the population and those which adopt a binary division based on social exclusion. The *politics stream* consists of interest groups, power bases and political cycles. Policies to tackle health inequalities are compatible with the government's political vision; however, departmental priorities and pressures may act against this (Gray and Jenkins, 2001; Flinders,

Table 6.1: Stages in health inequalities policy development

Stage	Selected examples of policies
Nature and extent of problem	Independent Inquiry into Inequalities in Health, 1998
Broad policy developments required	Government interventions in deprived areas, *2000 Spending Review* (HM Treasury, 2000)
	A new commitment to neighbourhood renewal (SEU, 2001)
	DoH *Consultation on a plan for delivery* (DoH, 2001b)
	2002 Spending Review (HM Treasury, 2002)
Public services response required to both improve health and reduce health inequalities	*Saving lives: Our healthier nation* (DoH, 1999a)
	Government interventions in deprived areas, *2000 Spending Review* (HM Treasury, 2000)
	A new commitment to neighbourhood renewal (SEU, 2001)
	DoH *Consultation on a plan for delivery* (DoH, 2001b)
Implementation in the NHS	*The NHS Plan* (DoH, 2000)
	National Service Frameworks, 2000 onwards
	NHS Cancer Plan (DoH, 2000)
	Local modernisation review (DoH, 2000)
Action and targets across government departments	PSAs (1998 and 2002)
	Opportunity for all (DSS, 1997)
	Government interventions in deprived areas, *2000 Spending Review* (HM Treasury, 2000)
	A new commitment to neighbourhood renewal (SEU, 2001)
	DoH *Consultation on a plan for delivery* (DoH, 2001b)
	2002 Spending Review (HM Treasury, 2002)
Trailblazer initiatives which contribute to reducing health inequalities	Health Action Zones and other action zones
	Sure Start programme
	New Deal for Communities
	PSA pilots
	Neighbourhood Management Pathfinders
	Healthy Living Centres
Mainstream planning processes and plans for local delivery of targets across the NHS and local government	LSPs
	HImPs
	Ministerial committee (overseeing Delivery Plan)
Mechanisms for monitoring targets	Neighbourhood Renewal Unit
	Basket of cross-government indicators
	NHS Performance assessment framework
	PSS Performance assessment framework
	Best Value performance indicators

Source: Adapted from Bull and Hamer (2001, pp 34-6)

2002). Two terms of office have enabled the government to devise and implement a longer-term, more coherent strategy than otherwise might be possible. This has been aided by a relatively favourable economic context (enabling some fiscal redistribution).

Table 6.2: Tackling health inequalities: a summary of progress (summer 2002)

Tackling health inequalities	Progress
1 Evidence of health inequalities – the nature of the 'problem'	Independent Inquiry, research and other evidence
2 Securing 'health inequalities' on the policy agenda	Widespread – not yet universal at national or local levels
3 Development of policies to tackle health inequalities	Diverse range of activity; increasing coherence
4 Implementation of initiatives	Current, ongoing
5 Integration into mainstream policy, planning and provision	Beginning
6 Intermediate markers/output indicators of policy implementation	Starting to emerge; health inequalities impact assessment still rare
7 Health outcomes (related to policy interventions)	Not yet apparent

However, the policy window cannot be guaranteed to remain open. Further progress in tackling health inequalities may be hampered by internal and external factors. Internal factors might include:

- lack of evidence of the effectiveness of policy interventions to tackle health inequalities;
- evidence of widening health inequalities;
- changes in health inequalities that cannot be attributed to specific policies.

External factors might include:

- wider socioeconomic context (such as persistent income inequalities);
- the dominance of healthcare (mainly NHS waiting lists and finances);
- other policies (such as road-building);
- the machinery of government itself (such as departmentalism or staff turnover).

The government's approach has opened the 'policy window' but we cannot, however, be complacent about whether it will necessarily remain open.

Substantial progress has been made but challenges remain. There are, however, indications that the government recognises the next stages of development. These include:

- introducing robust structures and processes for implementing policies;
- introducing effective performance management and monitoring systems to monitor such policies;
- embedding policies to tackle health inequalities within mainstream policy, planning and provision.

Many challenges remain but the prospects for tackling health inequalities are good.

7

Recommendations

The three primary recommendations of this report are supported by 15 subsidiary recommendations. Recommendations are linked to relevant sections in each chapter.

To central government

Introduce mechanisms that promote and ensure progress in policies to tackle health inequalities

Inequalities and Public Health Taskforce

1. Revise the role of the Inequalities and Public Health Taskforce to examine and promote ways in which a health inequality dimension can be embedded in 'mainstream' policy, planning and provision at central government and at the local level. (See page 48.)

Ministerial Sub-Committee on Social Exclusion (DA(SER))

2. Amend the terms of reference of the DA(SER) to include tackling health inequalities, and produce a rolling programme of work including tax and benefit policies. (See pages 22, 33 and 44.)
3. Create either a unit consisting of officials drawn from relevant departments or a clearly identified group of officials from those departments who work together to exchange information and produce material for the Inter-Ministerial Group on health inequalities. (See page 46.)
4. Commission the unit supporting the DA(SER) to:

- track progress on tackling health inequalities as identified during the monitoring of the relevant departmental PSAs and targets and the basket of indicators;
- advise on further action (such as the addition of new targets and objectives);
- act as a source of information and advice to departments on the data available both to assess the impact on health inequalities of policy proposals and for health inequalities impact assessments.
(See pages 24 and 33.)

5. Require the DA(SER) to produce an annual progress report for Parliament on tackling health inequalities. (See page 33.)
6. Form a special cross-departmental Select Committee (perhaps on an experimental basis initially), drawn from relevant departmental Select Committees in order to receive the annual report and to question Ministers on it. (See page 33.)

Data quality and availability

7. Ensure that departments are required to share relevant data on (a) inequalities in access to services in order to aid policy, planning and provision and (b) progress in meeting targets that are relevant to health inequalities. (See pages 38 and 46.)
8. Commission a review of relevant data collection to ensure that existing sources cover all factors and groups which need to be monitored in relation to health inequalities, notably social class, birth registrations by lone parents and ethnicity. As a result of this review, take action to address limitations in these – either by changes to routine data

collections or by commissioning studies (perhaps on a periodical basis) to provide the necessary information. (See page 46.)

Monitoring and assessment

9. Establish a range of interim indicators which track progress in establishing structure and process as well as longer-term indicators to appraise outcomes. Many existing PSAs and targets are relevant to tackling health inequalities. Progress on these should be regularly brought together and monitored to assess their overall impact on health inequalities and the wider determinants. (See pages 33 and 41.)

10. Make greater and/or more sensitive application of health inequalities impact assessment (especially across central government) through, for example, developing methodology, improving skills and capacity, refining data collection, conducting assessments prior to implementation and changing the scope of performance management systems. (See pages 24 and 44.)

Create an independent and regular evaluation of progress of policies to tackle health inequalities (in terms of policies' impacts on individuals, intermediate markers of progress and targets)

11. Create a mechanism (possibly under the auspices of Select Committees or the Audit Commission) to scrutinise and independently evaluate the annual progress report on health inequalities which would report to Parliament (Recommendation 6). (See page 33.)

12. Introduce mechanisms to enable local authority scrutiny committees to include health inequalities within their remit. (See page 44.)

To agencies which fund research (including the DoH, HDA, ESRC and MRC)

Create a centre of expertise to conduct and collate studies that describe and explain effective interventions to tackle health inequalities

13. Commission research to fill gaps in evidence of effectiveness of policies that reduce health inequalities (including social interventions and outcomes studies). (See page 46.)

14. Consider creating a centre of expertise to conduct and collate studies that describe and explain effective interventions to tackle health inequalities. (See page 46.)

15. Convene a forum of funding agencies involved in health inequalities research in order to coordinate research programmes which are focused on outcomes (rather than causation, which is relatively well established). (See page 46.)

References

Acheson, D. (chair) (1998) *Independent Inquiry into Inequalities in Health*, London: The Stationery Office.

Barker, A., Byrne, I. and Veall, A. (1999) *Ruling by taskforce*, London: Politico's Publishing.

Benzeval, M., Taylor, J. and Judge, K. (2000) 'Evidence on the relationship between low income and poor health: is the government doing enough?', *Fiscal Studies*, vol 21, no 3, pp 375-99.

Berridge, V. and Blume, S. (eds) (2002) *Poor health*, London: Frank Cass.

Black, D. (chair) (1980) *Inequalities in health*, London: Penguin.

Brewer, M. and Gregg, P. (2001) *Eradicating child poverty in Britain: Welfare reform and children since 1997*, WP01/08, London: IFS.

Brewer, M., Clark, T. and Myck, M. (2001) *Credit where it's due? An assessment of the new tax credits*, Commentary No 86, London: IFS.

Bull, J. and Hamer, L. (2001) *Closing the gap: Setting local targets to reduce health inequalities*, London: Health Development Agency.

Cabinet Office (2000) *Report of Policy Action Team 17: Joining it up locally*, London: Cabinet Office.

Cabinet Office/HM Treasury (2002) *Wiring it up: A progress report to the Prime Minister*, London: Cabinet Office/HM Treasury.

CASE (Centre for Analysis of Social Exclusion) (2000) *How effective is the British government's attempt to reduce child poverty?*, CASE Brief 15, London: London School of Economics and Political Science.

Catalyst Trust (2002) 'Response to the 2002 Budget', www.catalyst-trust.co.uk, April.

CPAG (Child Poverty Action Group) (2001) *An end in sight? Tackling child poverty in the UK*, London: CPAG.

Crombie, H. (2002) *The impact of transport and road traffic speed on health*, London: Health Development Agency.

Davies, H.T.O., Nutley, S. and Smith, P.C. (eds) (2000) *What works? Evidence-based policy and practice in public services*, Bristol: The Policy Press.

DEFRA (Department for Environment, Food and Rural Affairs) (2002) *Achieving a better quality of life: Review of progress towards sustainable development*, Government Annual Report 2001, London: DEFRA.

DETR (Department for the Environment, Transport and the Regions) (1998) *A New Deal for Transport: Better for everyone*, London: DETR.

DETR (2000) *Social exclusion and the provision and availability of public transport*, London: DETR.

DETR (2001a) *Older people: Their transport needs and requirements*, London: DETR.

DETR (2001b) *Road accident involvement of children from ethnic minorities: A literature review*, Road Safety Research Report No 19, London: DETR.

DfES (Department for Education and Skills) (nd) *Neighbourhood renewal: How DfES will meet its targets*, London: DfES.

DfES (2001) *Education and skills: Delivering results. A strategy to 2006*, London: DfES.

DfT (Department for Transport) (2001) *Transport statistics: Focus on personal travel*, London: DfT.

DfT (2002) *Road accidents Great Britain – The casualty report 2001*, London: DfT.

DoH (Department of Health) (1992) *Health of the nation*, London: HMSO.

DoH (1998a) 'Government committed to the greatest ever reduction in health inequalities, says Dobson', Press Release 98/547, 26 November.

DoH (1998b) *Our healthier nation: A contract for health*, London: The Stationery Office.

DoH (1999a) *Saving lives: Our healthier nation*, London: The Stationery Office.

DoH (1999b) *Action report on health inequalities*, London: DoH.

DoH (2000) *The NHS Plan*, London: DoH.

DoH (2001a) *From vision to reality*, London: DoH.

DoH (2001b) *Tackling health inequalities: Consultation on a plan for delivery*, London: DoH.

DoH (2001c) *Shifting the balance of power*, London: DoH.

DoH (2001d) 'Health inequalities: national targets on infant mortality and life expectancy – technical briefing. Infant mortality inequalities target – progress note', November, London: DoH.

DoH (2001e) *NHS performance indicators: A consultation*, London: DoH.

DoH (2001f) *Priorities and planning framework 2002/2003*, London: DoH.

DoH (2002a) *Tackling health inequalities: Update*, London: DoH.

DoH (2002b) *Tackling health inequalities: The results of the consultation exercise*, London: DoH.

DoH (2002c) *The years of life lost index and the health inequalities adjustment*, London: DoH.

DoH (2002d) *The next 3 years priorities and planning framework 2003-2006: Improvement, expansion and reform*, London: DoH.

DoH (2002e) 'NHS performance indicators: national figures', February, www.doh.gov.uk/nhsperformanceindicators/hlpi2002/ha-main.html.

DSS (Department of Social Security) (1997) *Opportunity for all – Tackling poverty and social exclusion: First annual report*, London: DSS.

DTLR (Department for Transport, Local Government and the Regions) (2000) *Tomorrow's roads: Safer for everyone. The government's road safety strategy and casualty reduction targets for 2010*, London: DTLR.

DTLR (2001a) *Strong local leadership – Quality public services*, White Paper, London: The Stationery Office.

DTLR (2001b) *Travel Concessions (Eligibility) Bill: Impact assessment*, London: DTLR.

DTLR (2001c) *Child pedestrian fatality figures for 2001*, London: DTLR.

DTLR (2002) 'Survey of concessionary bus fares: England 2001', News release 2002/0139, 28 March.

DTLR/DfES/DoH (2002) 'School travel', www.local-transport.dtlr.gov.uk/schooltravel/, April.

DWP (Department for Work and Pensions) (nd) 'Health and work policy and health inequalities', London: DWP.

DWP (2001) *Opportunity for all: The third annual report*, London: DWP.

DWP (2002a) *Opportunity for all: Fourth annual report*, London: DWP.

DWP (2002b) *Measuring child poverty: A consultation document*, London: DWP.

DWP (2002c) *Households below average income*, London: DWP.

Exworthy, M. (2002) 'The second Black Report? The Acheson Report as another opportunity to tackle health inequalities', in V. Berridge and S. Blume (eds) *Poor health*, London: Frank Cass, pp 175-97.

Exworthy, M. and Powell, M. (2000) 'Variations on a theme: New Labour, health inequalities and policy failure', in A. Hann (ed) *Analyzing health policy*, Aldershot: Ashgate, pp 45-62.

Exworthy, M., Berney, L. and Powell, M. (2002) 'How great expectations in Westminster may be dashed locally: the local implementation of national policy on health inequalities', *Policy & Politics*, vol 30, no 1, pp 79-96.

Flinders, A. (2002) 'Governance in Whitehall', *Public Administration*, vol 80, no 1, pp 51-75.

Graham, H. (ed) (2000) *Understanding health inequalities*, Buckingham: Open University Press.

Gray, A. and Jenkins, B. (2001) 'Government and administration: the dilemmas of delivery', *Parliamentary Affairs*, vol 54, pp 206-22.

HDA (Health Development Agency) (1998) *Transport and health: A briefing for health professionals and local authorities*, London: HDA.

HDA (2002) *Performance managing public health action in primary care trusts: A briefing for chief executives of strategic health authorities*, London: HDA.

HM Treasury (1999) *The modernisation of Britain's tax and benefit system: Number four: tackling poverty and extending opportunity*, London: HM Treasury.

HM Treasury (2000) *2000 Spending Review: Public service agreements*, Cmd 4808, London: The Stationery Office.

HM Treasury (2001a) *Building a stronger, fairer Britain in an uncertain world: Pre-Budget report 2001*, London: HM Treasury.

HM Treasury (2001b) 'Andrew Smith sets out priorities for 2002 Spending Review', Press release 72/01, 25 June.

HM Treasury (2002) *2002 Spending Review: Opportunity and security for all: investing for an enterprising, fairer Britain. New public spending plans 2003-2006*, London: The Stationery Office.

HM Treasury/DoH (2002) *Tackling inequalities: Summary of the 2002 Cross-cutting Review*, London: HM Treasury.

IFS (Institute for Fiscal Studies) (2000) *Responses to the Budget*, London: IFS.

IFS (2002) *Responses to the Budget*, London: IFS.

JRF (Joseph Rowntree Foundation) (2001) 'Environment and equity concerns about transport', Findings 721, York: Joseph Rowntree Foundation.

Kingdon, J. (1995) *Agendas, alternatives and public policy*, 2nd edn, New York, NY: Harper Collins.

Laflamme, L. and Engstrom, K. (2002) 'Socio-economic differences in Swedish children and adolescents injured in road traffic accidents: a cross-sectional study', *British Medical Journal*, vol 324, pp 396-7.

London Health Commission (2001) *A report of a health impact assessment of the Mayor's draft transport strategy by the London Health Commission*, September, London: London Health Commission.

Maddock, S. (2000) *Mainstreaming: Learning from the Health Action Zones*, Manchester: Manchester Business School.

Marmot, M. (1999) 'Acting on the evidence to reduce inequalities in health', *Health Affairs*, vol 18, no 3, May/June, pp 42-4.

Marmot, M. and Wilkinson, R.G. (eds) (1999) *Social determinants of health*, Oxford: Oxford University Press.

NAO (National Audit Office) (2001a) *Joining it up to improve public services*, HC383, 2001-02, London: NAO.

NAO (2001b) *Policy development: Improving air quality*, HC232, 2001-02, London: NAO.

National Statistics (2002) 'Households below average income statistics', first release 11 April.

ONS (Office for National Statistics) (2000) *The effect of taxes and benefits on household income, 1998-1999*, London: ONS.

ONS (2001) *The effect of taxes and benefits on household income, 1999-2000*, London: ONS.

ONS (2002) *The effects of taxes and benefits on household incomes, 2000-2001*, at www.statistics.gov.uk.

Paull, G., Taylor, J. and Duncan, A. (2002) *Mothers' employment and childcare use in the UK*, London: IFS.

PIU (Performance and Innovation Unit) (2000) *Wiring it up: Whitehall's management of cross-cutting policies and services*, London: Cabinet Office.

Powell, M. (ed) (1999) *New Labour, new welfare state? The 'third way' in British social policy*, Bristol: The Policy Press.

Powell, M. and Exworthy, M. (2001) 'Joined-up solutions to address health inequalities: analysing policy, process and resources streams', *Public Money and Management*, vol 21, no 4, pp 21-6.

Richards, D. and Smith, M.J. (2002) 'The paradoxes of policy co-ordination: Britain – a case-study of joined-up government', Paper presented to the Structure and Organisation of Government International conference, Melbourne University, Australia, 3-5 June.

Richards, S. (2001) 'Four types of joined up government and the problem of accountability', in NAO, *Joining it up to improve public services*, HC383, 2001-02, London: NAO, pp 61-70.

Scottish Office (1999) *Towards a healthier Scotland – A White Paper*, Cmd 4269, February, Edinburgh: Scottish Office.

SEU (Social Exclusion Unit) (2001) *A new commitment to neighbourhood renewal: National strategy action plan*, London: SEU.

SEU (2002) *Making the connections: Transport and social exclusion*, London: SEU.

Shaw, M., Dorling, D., Gordon, D. and Davey Smith, G. (2001) 'Health', in G. Finnister (ed) *An end in sight? Tackling child poverty in the UK*, London: CPAG.

Smith, P.C. (2002) 'Performance management in British health care: will it deliver?', *Health Affairs*, vol 21, no 3, May/June, pp 103-15.

Stewart, M., Grimshaw, L., Purdue, D., May, A., Carlton, N., Goss, S., Gillanders, G., Courage, S., Albury, D., Cowley, C., Thompson, H. and Dixon, R., with Cameron, S., Coaffee, J., Merridew, T., Healey, P. and de Magalhes, C. (2002) *Collaboration and coordination in area based initiatives*, Research Report No 1, London: ODPM.

Sure Start (nd(a)) 'Sure Start's Public Service Agreement 2001-04: technical note', London: DfES.

Sure Start (nd(b)) 'Service delivery agreement', London: DfES.

Sure Start (2000) *Sure Start and services for the under 5s: A report for the 2000 Spending Review*, London: DfES.

Sure Start (2001a) *A guide to planning and running your programme*, London: DfES.

Sure Start (2001b) *A guide for fifth wave programmes*, London: DfES.

Wanless, D. (2002) *Securing our future health: Taking a long-term view: Final report*, London: DoH.

Appendix A:
Advisory Group membership

The project team was supported by an Advisory Group, which met five times during the course of the project (February 2001 to September 2002).

Sir Donald Acheson	University College London
Dr David Blane	Imperial College London
Dr Jacky Chambers	Heart of Birmingham (teaching) PCT
Dr Mark Exworthy	University College London
Norman Glass	National Centre for Social Research
Donald Hirsch	Joseph Rowntree Foundation
Professor Mike Kelly	Health Development Agency
Pat Kneen	Joseph Rowntree Foundation
Dr Catherine Law	Southampton University
Professor Sir Michael Marmot	University College London
Professor Steve Platt	Edinburgh University
Edna Robinson	Trafford South PCT
Marian Stuart	Project adviser
Professor Margaret Whitehead	University of Liverpool

B

Appendix B: Membership of the Independent Inquiry into Inequalities in Health (1997-98)

The membership comprised:

Sir Donald Acheson (Chair)	University College London
Professor David Barker	Southampton University
Dr Jacky Chambers	Birmingham Health Authority
Frances Drever (Statistical Adviser)	Office for National Statistics
Ray Earwicker (Administrative Secretary)	Department of Health
Professor Hilary Graham	Lancaster University
Dr Catherine Law (Scientific Secretary)	Southampton University
Professor Michael Marmot	University College London
Professor Margaret Whitehead	University of Liverpool

An evaluation group was established to examine the quality of the evidence underpinning the group's recommendations. The evaluation group comprised:

Professor Sally Macintyre	Glasgow University
Ian Chalmers	Cochrane Centre, Oxford
Richard Horton	Editor, *Lancet*
Richard Smith	Editor, *British Medical Journal*

Appendix C: Independent Inquiry (Acheson Report) main recommendations

1. All policies likely to have [an] effect on health should be evaluated in terms of their impact on health inequalities and [policies] should be formulated in such a way that by favouring the less well off, they will ... reduce such inequalities.

2. A high priority is given to policies aimed at improving health and reducing health inequalities in women of childbearing age, expectant mothers and young children.

3. Policies which will further reduce income inequalities and improve the living standards of households in receipt of social security benefits.

4. Provision of additional resources for schools serving children from less well off groups to enhance their educational achievement. The RSG formula and other funding mechanism should be more strongly weighted to reflect need and socio-economic disadvantage.

5. Further development of high quality pre-school education so that it meets, in particular, the needs of disadvantaged families. Benefits or pre-school education to disadvantaged families are evaluated and, if necessary, additional resources are made available to support further development.

6. Further development of 'health promoting schools', initially focused on, but not limited to, disadvantaged communities.

7. Further measures to improve the nutrition provided at school, including: the promotion of school food policies, the development of budgeting and cooking skills, the preservation of free school meals entitlement, the provision of free school fruit and the restriction of less health[y?] food.

8. Policies which improve the opportunities for work and which ameliorate the health consequences of unemployment.

9. Policies which improve the quality of jobs and reduce psychosocial work hazards.

10. Policies which improve the availability of social housing for the less well off within a framework of environmental improvement, planning and design which takes into account social networks and access to goods and services.

11. Policies which improve housing provision and access to health care for homeless people.

12. Policies which aim to improve the quality of housing.

13. The development of policies to reduce the fear of crime and violence and to create a safe environment for people to live in.

14. Further development of a high quality public transport system which is integrated with other forms of transport and is affordable to the user.

15. Further measures to encourage walking and cycling as forms of transport and to ensure the safe separation of pedestrians and cyclists from motor vehicles.

16. Further steps to reduce the usage of motor cars to cut the mortality and morbidity associated with motor vehicle emissions.

17. Further measures to reduce traffic speeds, by environmental design, and modifications of roads, lower speed limits in built up areas and stricter enforcement of speed limits.

18. Concessionary fares should be available to pensioners and disadvantaged groups throughout the country and that local schemes should emulate high quality schemes.

19. A comprehensive review of the Common Agricultural Policy's impact on health and inequalities in health.

20. Policies which will increase the availability and accessibility of foodstuffs to supply an adequate and affordable diet.

21. Policies which reduce poverty in families with children by promoting the material support of parents; by removing barriers to work for parents who wish to combine work with parenting, and by enabling those who wish to do so to devote full-time to parenting to do so.

22. Policies which improve the health and nutrition of women of childbearing age and their children with priority given to the elimination of food poverty and the prevention and reduction of obesity.

23. Policies that promote the social and emotional support for parent children.

24. Measures to prevent suicide among young people especially young men and seriously mentally ill young people.

25. Policies which promote sexual health in young people and reduce unwanted teenage pregnancy including access to appropriate contraceptive services.

26. Policies which promote the adoption of healthier lifestyles, particularly in respect of factors which show a strong social gradient in prevalence or consequences.

27. Policies which will promote the material well being of older people.

28. Quality of homes in which older people live be improved.

29. Policies which will promote the maintenance of mobility, independence and social contacts.

30. Further development of health and social services for older people, so that these services are accessible and distributed according to need.

31. Further development of services which are sensitive to the needs of minority ethnic groups and which promote greater awareness of their health risks.

32. Needs of minority ethnic groups are specifically considered in needs assessment, resource allocation, health care planning and provision.

33. Needs of minority ethnic groups are specifically considered in needs assessment, resource allocation, health care planning and provision.

34. Policies which reduce the excess mortality from accidents and suicide in young men.

35. Policies which reduce psychosocial ill-health in young women in disadvantaged circumstances particularly those caring for young children.

36. Policies which reduce disability and ameliorate its consequence in older women, particularly those living alone.

37. Providing equitable access to effective care in relation to need should be a governing principle of all policies in the NHS. Priority should be given to the achievement of equity in planning, implementation and delivery of services at every level of the NHS.

38. Giving priority to the achievement of a more equitable allocation of NHS resources. This will require adjustments to the ways in which resources are allocated and the speed with which resource allocation targets are met.

39. Directors of Public Health, working on behalf of HA and LA, produce an equity profile for the population they serve and undertake a triennial audit of progress towards achieving objectives to reduce inequalities in health.

Appendix D:
Targets for tackling
health inequalities

National health inequality targets (2001)

Starting with children under one year, by 2010, to reduce by at least 10% the gap in mortality between manual groups and the population as a whole.

Starting with health authorities, by 2010, to reduce by at least 10% the gap between the fifth of areas with the lowest life expectancy at birth and the population as a whole.

Teenage conception rate target (2001)

By achieving agreed local conception reduction targets, to reduce the national under-18 conception rate by 15% by 2004, and 50% by 2010 while reducing the gap in rates between the worst fifth of [electoral] wards and the average by at least a quarter.

Smoking reduction/cessation targets

To reduce smoking rates among manual groups from 32% to 26% by 2010.

By 2010, reduce cancer mortality rates by more than 20% in people under 75 by 2010, aiming to improve the health of the worst off in particular (NHS Cancer Plan, 2000).

To achieve a 10% reduction in the number of mothers who smoke during pregnancy in the 500 Sure Start areas by 2004.

Saving lives: Our healthier nation White Paper targets (1999)

Heart disease and stroke

To reduce the death rate in people under 75 by at least two fifths.

Accidents

To reduce the death rate by at least a fifth and serious injury by at least a tenth.

Cancer

To reduce the death rate in people under 75 by at least a fifth.

Mental health

To reduce the death rate from suicide and undetermined injury by at least a fifth.

Educational attainment target

To ensure no school has fewer than 25% of pupils getting five good GCSE passes by 2004.

To increase the proportion of 11-year-olds reaching the expected standard for their age to 80% for literacy and 75% for numeracy by 2002 (DWP, 2001, p 45).

To reduce number of adults with literacy and numeracy problems by 750,000 by 2004.

Child poverty target (DWP PSA, 2002)

To reduce the number of children living in low-income households by at least a quarter by 2004, as a contribution towards the broader target of halving child poverty by 2010 and eradicating it by 2020.

Housing-related targets

To reduce the number of people sleeping rough in England by at least two thirds between June 1998 and April 2002.

To bring all social housing up to a decent standard within 10 years.

To reduce the number of households in social housing that does not meet standards by a third, 2001-04.

To reduce fuel poverty in vulnerable households by improving the energy efficiency of 600,000 homes.

Crime reduction target

To reduce crime, including domestic burglary by 25% by 2005.

Transport targets

To reduce the number of people killed or seriously injured by 40% and the number of children killed or seriously injured by 50%, by 2010 compared with the 1994-98 average.

To meet EU vehicle emission standards and fuel quality standards from 2000.

Early years targets

To close the gap between the availability of accessible childcare for 0- to 3-year-olds.

To close the childcare gap between Sure Start areas and other areas.

To reduce the proportion of children (aged 0-3) in the 500 Sure Start areas who are registered within the space of 12 months on the child protection register, by 20% by 2004.

Employment target

To ensure that 70% of lone parents are in employment by 2010.

Neighbourhood Renewal targets (ODPM)

To eliminate substandard social housing by 2010, and reduce it by a third by 2004.

To ensure no area has burglary rates three times higher than the national average by 2004.

To ensure at least 25% of pupils in every school and 38% in every local authority area achieve five or more GCSEs at grades A* to C.

Starting with health authorities, by 2010, to reduce by at least 10% the gap between the quintile of areas with the lowest life expectancy at birth and the population as a whole.

To reduce by at least 60%, by 2010, the conception rate among under-18s in the worst 20% of wards, and thereby reduce the level of inequality between these areas and the average by at least 26% by 2010.

To raise the employment in the 30 local districts with the worst labour market problems and to narrow the gap between these and the overall rate.

DEFRA sustainable development indicators

- Success in tackling poverty and social exclusion
- Homes judged unfit to live in
- Proportion of people of working age out of work for more than two years
- People in employment working long hours
- Working fatalities and injury rates
- Working days lost through illness
- Pesticide residue in foods
- Index of local deprivation

- Truancies and exclusions from school/ teenage pregnancy
- How children get to school
- Access to services in rural areas
- Participation in sport and cultural activities
- Fear of crime
- Concentrations of persistent organic pollutants
- Dangerous substances in water
  Source: DEFRA (2002)

Public Service Agreements

PSAs are discussed in Chapter 4. The PSAs that have particular relevance to health inequalities cover the following departments:

- Department of Health
- Department for Education and Skills
- Department for Transport
- Home Office
- Department for Environment, Food and Rural Affairs
- Department for Culture, Media and Sport
- Department for Work and Pensions
- HM Treasury
- Sure Start, early years and childcare

Department of Health: selected PSAs (2002)

Aim

Transform the health and social care system so that it produces faster, fairer services that deliver better health and tackle health inequalities.

Objective I: Improve service standards

1. Reduce the maximum wait for an outpatient appointment to three months ... by the end of 2005.
2. Reduce to four hours the maximum wait in A&E ... by the end of 2004.
3. Guarantee access to a primary care professional within 24 hours.
4. Ensure that by the end of 2005 every hospital appointment will be booked for the convenience of the patient.
5. Enhance accountability to patients.

Objective II: Improve health and social care outcomes for everyone

6. Reduce substantially the mortality rates from the major killer diseases by 2010.
7. Improve life outcomes of adults and children with mental health problems ... and reduce the mortality rate from suicide and undetermined injury by at least 20% by 2010.
8. Improve the quality of life and independence of older people.
9. Improve the life chances for children by improving the level of education, training and employment outcomes for care leavers ..., narrowing the gap between the proportions of children in care and their peers who are cautioned or convicted, and reducing the under-18 conception rate by 50% by 2010.
10. Increase the participation of problem drug users in drug treatment programmes.
11. By 2010, reduce inequalities in health outcomes by 10% as measured by infant mortality and life expectancy at birth.

Department for Education and Skills: selected PSAs (2002)

Objective I: Sustain improvements in primary education

1. Raise standards in English and maths ... by 2004 and 2007.

Objective II: Transform secondary education

2. Raise standards in English, maths, ICT and science in secondary education ... by 2004 and 2007.

Objective III: Pupil inclusion

3. By 2004 reduce school truancies by 10% compared to 2002.
4. Enhance the take-up of sporting opportunities by 5- to 16-year-olds.

Objective IV: Raise attainment at 14-19

5. Raise standards in schools and colleges.

Objective V: Improve the skills of young people and adults and raise participation and quality in post-16 learning provision

Objective VI: Tackle the adult skills deficit

Department for Transport: selected PSAs (2002)

Aim

Transport that works for everyone.

Objective I: Reliable, safe and secure transport for everyone which respects the environment

1. Reduce congestion on the inter-urban road networks ... by 2010.
2. Secure improvements in rail punctuality and reliability with a 50% increase in rail use from 2000 levels by 2010.
3. Secure improvements in the accessibility, punctuality and reliability of local public transport, with an increase in use of more than 12% by 2010 compared with 2000 levels.
4. Cut journey times on London Underground.
5. Reduce the number of people killed or seriously injured in Great Britain in road accidents by 40% and the number of children killed or seriously injured by 50%, by 2010 compared with the average for 1994-98, tackling the significantly higher incidence in disadvantaged communities.
6. Improve air quality by meeting our National Air Quality strategy objectives.

Home Office: selected PSAs (2002)

Aim

To build a safe, just and tolerant society.

Objective 1: Reduce crime and the fear of crime

1. Reduce crime and the fear of crime; improve performance overall, including by reducing the gap between the highest Crime and Disorder Reduction Partnership areas and the best comparable areas; and reduce vehicle crime by 30% from 1998-99 to 2004; domestic burglary by 25% from 1998-99 to 2005, robbery in the 10 Street Crime Initiative areas by 14% from 1999-2000 to 2005.
2. Improve the performance of all police forces and significantly reduce the performance gap between the best and worst performing forces, and significantly increase the proportion of time spent on frontline duties.

Objective II: Ensure the effective delivery of justice

3. Improve the delivery of justice by increasing the number of crimes for which an offender is brought to justice by 1.2 million by 2005-06; with an improvement in all Criminal Justice System areas, a greater increase in the worst performing areas and a reduction in the proportion of ineffective trials.
4. Improve the level of public confidence in the Criminal Justice System, including increasing that of ethnic minority communities, and increasing year-on-year the satisfaction of victims and witnesses, while respecting the rights of defendants.

Objective VI: Support strong and active communities in which people of all races and backgrounds are valued and participate on equal terms

8. Increase voluntary and community sector activity, including community participation by 5% by 2006.
9. Bring about measurable improvements in race equality and community cohesion across a range of performance indicators, as part of the government's objectives on equality and social inclusion.

Department for Environment, Food and Rural Affairs: selected PSAs (2002)

Aim

Sustainable development, which means a better quality of life for everyone, now and for generations to come, including a better environment at home and internationally, and sustainable use of natural resources.

Objectives

Promote sustainable development across government and the country as a whole as measured by achieving positive trends in the government's headline indicators of sustainable development.

Objective I: Protect and improve the rural, urban, marine and global environment, and lead integration of these with other policies across Government and internationally

Objective II: Enhance opportunity and tackle social exclusion in rural areas

4. Reduce the gap in productivity between the least well performing quartile of rural areas and the English median by 2006, and improve the accessibility of services for rural people.

Objective III: Promote a sustainable, competitive and safe food supply chain, which meets consumers' requirements

Objective IV: Promote sustainable, diverse, modern and adaptable farming through domestic and international actions

5. Deliver more customer-focused, competitive and sustainable food and farming...; and secure CAP reforms that reduce production-linked support, enabling enhanced EU funding for environmental conservation and rural development.

Objective V: Promote sustainable management and prudent use of natural resources domestically and internationally.

6. Enable 25% of household waste to be recycled or composted by 2005-06.
7. Reduce fuel poverty among vulnerable households by improving the energy efficiency of 600,000 homes between 2001 and 2004.

Objective VI: Protect the public's interest in relation to environmental impacts and health, and ensure high standards of animal health and welfare.

8. Improve air quality by meeting our National Air Quality Strategy objectives for carbon monoxide, lead, nitrogen dioxide, particles, sulphur dioxide, benzene and 1-3 butadiene.

Department of Culture, Media and Sport: selected PSAs (2002)

Aim

Improve the quality of life for all through cultural and sporting activities, to support the pursuit of excellence and champion the tourism, creative and leisure industries.

Objective I: Increase participation in culture and sport and develop our sectors

1. Enhance the take-up of sporting opportunities by 5- to 16-year-olds by increasing the percentage of schoolchildren who spend a minimum of two hours each week on high quality PE and school sport within and beyond the curriculum from 25% in 2002 to 75% by 2006.
2. Increase significantly the take-up of cultural and sporting opportunities by new users aged 20 and above from priority groups.

Objective II: Develop appropriate regulatory frameworks that protect consumers' interests and improve the productivity of our sectors

Department for Work and Pensions: selected PSAs (2002)

Objective I: Ensure the best start for all children and end child poverty in 20 years

1. Reduce the number of children in low-income households by at least a quarter by 2004, as a contribution towards the broader target of halving child poverty by 2010 and eradicating it by 2020.

Objective II: Promote work as the best form of welfare for people of working age, while protecting the position of those in greatest need

3. Demonstrate progress by spring 2006 on increasing the employment and reducing the unemployment rate over the economic cycle.
4. Over the three years to 2006, increase the employment rates of disadvantaged areas and groups ... and significantly reduce the difference between their employment rates and the overall rate.

5. Reduce the proportion of children in households with no one in work over the three years from spring 2003 to spring 2006 by 6½%.

Objective III: Combat poverty and promote security and independence in retirement for today's and tomorrow's pensioners

Objective IV: Improve rights and opportunities for disabled people in a fair and inclusive society

7. Over the three years to 2006, increase the employment rate of people with disabilities ... and significantly reduce the difference between their employment rates and the overall rate.

Objective V: Modernise welfare delivery so as to improve the accessibility, accuracy and value for money of services to customers including employers

HM Treasury: selected PSAs (2002)

Aim

Raise the rate of sustainable growth and achieve rising prosperity and a better quality of life, with economic and employment opportunities for all.

Objective I: Maintain a stable macroeconomic framework with low inflation

Objective II: Maintain sound public finances in accordance with the Code for Fiscal Stability

Objective III: Promote UK economic prospects by pursuing increased productivity and efficiency in the EU, international financial stability and increased global prosperity, including especially protecting the most vulnerable.

4. Promote increased global prosperity and social justice.

Objective IV: Increase the productivity of the economy

6. Make sustainable improvements in the economic performance of all English regions and, over the long term, reduce the persistent gap in growth rates between the regions,

defining measures to improve performance and reporting progress against these measures by 2006.

Objective VI: Expand economic and employment opportunities for all

7. Demonstrate progress by Spring 2006 on increasing the employment rate and reducing the unemployment rate over the economic cycle.

Objective VII: Promote a fair and efficient tax and benefit system with incentives to work, save and invest

8. Reduce the number of children in low-income households by at least a quarter by 2004, as a contribution towards the broader target of halving child poverty by 2010 and eradicating it by 2020. Joint target with DWP.

Objective VIII: Improve the quality and the cost effectiveness of public services

9. Improve public services by working with departments to help them meet their PSA targets, consistently with the fiscal rules.

Sure Start, early years and childcare: PSAs (2002)

Performance targets

1. In fully operational programmes, achieve by 2005-06:
- an increase in the proportion of young children aged 0-5 with normal levels of personal, social and emotional development for their age;
- a six percentage point reduction in the proportion of mothers who continue to smoke during pregnancy;
- an increase in the proportion of children having normal levels of communication, language and literacy;
- a 12% reduction in the proportion of young children living in households where no one is working.

A decision will be taken shortly on the Ministerial responsibilities for the unit.

Source: HM Treasury (2002)
Welfare-to-Work had a (cross-cutting) PSA in 2000 but not in 2002.